THE EXECUTIVE BRAIN

THE EXECUTIVE BRAIN

FRONTAL LOBES AND THE CIVILIZED MIND

Elkhonon Goldberg

OXFORD
UNIVERSITY PRESS

OXFORD
UNIVERSITY PRESS

Oxford New York
Auckland Bangkok Buenos Aires
Cape Town Chennai Dar es Salaam Delhi Hong Kong Istanbul
Karachi Kolkata Kuala Lumpur Madrid Melbourne Mexico City Mumbai
Nairobi São Paulo Shanghai Singapore Taipei Tokyo Toronto

and an associated company in Berlin

First published by Oxford University Press, Inc., 2001
198 Madison Avenue, New York, New York, 10016
First issued as an Oxford University Press paperback, 2002

Library of Congress Cataloging-in-Publication Data
Goldberg, Elkhonon.
The executive brain : frontal lobes and the civilized mind/
Elkhonon Goldberg.
p. cm.
Includes bibliographical references and index.
ISBN 0-19-514022-2 (cloth) ISBN 0-19-515630-7 (pbk.)
1. Frontal lobes. 2. Neuropsychology. I. Title.
QP382.F7 G65 2001 612.8'25—dc21 00-058447

1 3 5 7 9 10 8 6 4 2

Printed in the United States of America
on acid-free paper

To my teacher Alexandr Luria,
who sparked the interest that led
to this book

Foreword

Oliver Sacks

In 1967, Elkhonon Goldberg, then a twenty-year-old student of neuropsychology in Moscow, met a young man, another student only a few years older than himself. Vladimir, Goldberg tells us, had been standing on the platform of the Moscow subway, tossing a soccer ball from hand to hand, when the ball fell onto the rails. Jumping down to retrieve it, Vladimir was hit by a train and sustained severe damage to the front part of the brain, the frontal lobes, both of which had to be amputated.

"The career of every clinician," Goldberg writes, "is punctuated by a few formative cases. Vladimir was my first formative case. Unwittingly, through his tragedy, he introduced me to the rich phenomena of frontal-lobe disease, triggered my interest in the frontal lobes, and so helped shape my career." While Vladimir spent most of his time staring blankly into space (though when disturbed he might release a stream of profanities or hurl a chamberpot), Goldberg found that he could sometimes engage him with "a casually profane, locker-room-style banter . . . [and] a friendship of sorts developed between a brain-damaged student and a student of brain damage."

Goldberg's mentor, the great Russian neuropsychologist A. R. Luria, was becoming increasingly interested in these "highest" parts of the brain, and suggested to Goldberg that their study might become his project too. This project has now lasted a third of a century, and has taken Goldberg into some of the profoundest and strangest realms of brain–mind functioning and its mishaps. Like

Luria, he has employed a mixture of specially tailored and ingenious tests with a minute naturalistic observation, alert to the vagaries of frontal lobe function not only in the clinic but in streets, in restaurants, in the theater, everywhere. (Goldberg speaks of himself here as a "cognitive voyeur.") All this is leavened with exceptional imaginative and empathic powers, trying to see the world through his patients' eyes. With thirty years of observation and experience, he has achieved a level of insight which, one feels, would have delighted and amazed his mentor, Luria.

In *The Executive Brain,* Goldberg takes us on a journey, his own journey, from those early Moscow days to the present, a journey at once intellectual and personal. He provides a brilliant exposition of the complex functions of the frontal lobes, this most recently evolved and especially human part of the brain, examining the great range of frontal lobe "styles" in normal people, the tragic mishaps which may occur with neurological disease or brain damage, the ways in which their function can be tested, and not least, the ways in which frontal lobe function can be strengthened—many of which Goldberg himself has pioneered—building or rebuilding cognitive function generally, not only in brain-damaged patients but in the healthy brain as well. (Goldberg's notion of "cognitive fitness" and the use of "cognitive exercise" and a "cognitive gym" are particularly challenging—and important.) Rich case histories, along with brief but revelatory neuropsychological anecdotes, form the narrative heart of the book, but they are frequently interleaved with personal narratives of every sort, and this makes *The Executive Brain* a highly engaging and intimate memoir, a sort of intellectual autobiography, no less than a grand piece of scientific reporting and "popular" science.

The Executive Brain is dedicated to Luria, and opens movingly with a memory of a conversation with Luria in 1972—Goldberg was 25 at the time, and Luria 70, at once his illustrious mentor and a most affectionate and supportive father figure. Luria pressed Goldberg to join the Communist Party, offering to nominate him, and underscoring the necessity of this for any career advancement in the Soviet Union. (Luria was himself a member of the Party, more from expedience, perhaps, than from conviction.) But Goldberg was (and remains) a rebel at heart, not disposed to make compromises, however advantageous, if they went against his inner instincts. Such instransigence was costly in the Soviet Union, and had landed his father in the Gulag. After prevaricating a dozen times, he finally told Luria outright that he would not join the Party. Further—though this, of course, he did not say—he had decided to leave Russia, despite a profound love for his motherland and language. It was virtually impossible for a highly valued member of society, a doctoral student at Moscow University, to leave the country, and Goldberg's narrative of how he did this, and in a way which would avoid compromising Luria in any way, forms the extraordinary and compelling introduction to this book, a book which ends 26 years later, with a return visit to Moscow and the country he left half a lifetime before.

The frontal lobes are the latest achievement in the evolution of the nervous system; it is only in human beings (and great apes, to some extent) that they reach so great a development. They were also, by a curious parallel, the last parts of the brain to be recognized as important—even in my own medical student days, they were called "the silent lobes." "Silent" indeed they may be, for they lack the simple and easily identifiable functions of the more primitive parts of the cerebral cortex, the sensory and motor areas, for example (and even the "association areas" between these), but they are overwhelmingly important. They are crucial for all higher-order purposeful behavior—identifying the objective, projecting the goal, forging plans to reach it, organizing the means by which such plans can be carried out, monitoring and judging the consequences to see that all is accomplished as intended.

This is the central role of the frontal lobes, one which releases the organism from fixed repertoires and reactions, allows the mental representation of alternatives, imagination, freedom. Thus the metaphors that run through the book: the frontal lobes as the brain's CEO, capable of taking "an aerial view" of all the other functions of the brain and coordinating them; the frontal lobes as the brain's conductor, coordinating the thousand instruments in the brain's orchestra. But above all, the frontal lobes as the brain's leader, leading the individual into the novelty, the innovations, the adventures of life. Without the great development of the frontal lobes in the human brain (coupled with the development of the language areas), civilization could never have arisen.

The intentionality of the individual is invested in the frontal lobes, and these are crucial for higher consciousness, for judgment, for imagination, for empathy, for identity, for "soul." Thus in the famous case of Phineas Gage—a railway foreman who while setting an explosive charge in 1848 had a two-foot tamping iron blown through his frontal lobes when the charge backfired—while there was preservation of Gage's intelligence as well as his ability to move and talk and see, there were other, profound changes in him. He became reckless and improvident, impulsive, profane; he could no longer plan or think of the future; and for those who had known him before, "he was no longer Gage." He had lost himself, the most central part of his being, and (as is the case with all patients with severe damage to the frontal lobes), he did not know it.

Such an "anosognosia," as it is called, is at once a mercy (such patients do not suffer or anguish or lament their loss), and a major problem, for it undercuts understanding and motivation, and makes attempts to remediate the condition much more difficult.

Goldberg also brings out how, because of the unique richness of the frontal lobes's connections to different parts of the brain, other conditions which have their primary pathology elsewhere, even in the subcortex, may evoke or present as frontal lobe dysfunctions. Thus the inertia of parkinsonism, the impulsiveness of Tourette's syndrome, the distractibility of ADHD, the perseveration of OCD, the lack of empathy or "theory of mind" in autism or chronic schizophrenia, can all be understood, in large part, Goldberg feels, as due to the resonances, the secondary disturbances, in the function of the frontal lobes. Much evidence is adduced in favor of this, not only from clinical observation and testing, but from the latest results in functional brain imaging, and Goldberg's insights here illuminate these syndromes in a new way, and may be very important in clinical practice.

While patients with massive frontal lobe lesions show an unawareness of their condition, this is not so for patients with parkinsonism, Tourette's syndrome, OCD, ADHD, or autism; indeed such patients can articulate and often analyze with great accuracy what is going on with them. Thus they can tell us what patients with primary frontal lobe pathology cannot—what it actually feels like from the inside to have these differences and vagaries of frontal lobe function.

Goldberg presents these discussions, which might otherwise be difficult or dense, with great vividness and humor, and with frequent alternations of personal narrative. Thus in the middle of his discussion of "field-dependent" behavior, the incontinent distractibility so characteristic of those with severe frontal lobe damage, Goldberg speaks of dogs, and their relatively "afrontal" behavior, where "out of sight" is "out of mind." He contrasts this with the behavior of apes, and tells us how, on a trip to Thailand, he once "befriended and was befriended by" a young male gibbon, the pet of a restaurant owner in Phuket:

> Every morning the gibbon rushed forth to shake hands. All limbs and a small body, he would then engage in a brief spider-like dance, which, in my self-flattering way, I interpreted as an expression of joy at seeing me. But then, despite his proclivity for restless play, he would settle next to me and with extreme concentration would study the minute details of my clothes: a watchband, a button, a shoe, my glasses (which, in one of my unguarded moments, he took off my face and tried for lunch). He stared at the items intently and systematically shifted his gaze from one detail to another. When one day a bandage appeared around my index finger, the young gibbon studiously examined it. Despite his status of a "lesser" ape (in contrast to the bonobos, chimpanzees, gorillas, and orangutans, which are known as the "great" apes), the gibbon was capable of sustained attention.
>
> Most remarkably, the gibbon invariably turned *back* to the object of his curiosity following a sudden distraction, say, a street noise. He would resume his exploration precisely where it had been interrupted, even when the interruption was more than a split second in length. The gibbon's actions were guided by an internal representation, which "bridged" his behavior beween before and after the distraction. "Out of sight" was no longer "out of mind"!

Goldberg is a dog lover, and has owned several dogs, but for him "the interaction with the gibbon was so qualitatively different from, and so strikingly richer than, anything I had ever experienced with dogs, that I briefly entertained the idea of buying the gibbon and bringing him to New York to be my pet and companion."

This, of course, was impossible, and Goldberg (whom I knew by this time) was very sad that he could not do so. I felt a great sympathy for him because I had had an almost identical experience with an orangutan myself, and had more than half-wished we could at least send postcards to each other.

■ ■ ■

There are other major themes in *The Executive Brain*, ideas which first surfaced when Goldberg was a student, and which he has been exploring and elaborating ever since. These have to do with the different sorts of challenge which face an organism: the encountering of novel situations (and the need to arrive at novel solutions), and the need to have set, economical routines for dealing with familiar situations and demands. Goldberg sees the right hemisphere of the brain as especially equipped to deal with novel situations and solutions, and the left side of the brain with routine tasks and processes. There is, in his view, a continual cycling of information, of understanding, from the right to the left hemisphere. "The transition from novelty to routinization," he writes, "is the universal cycle of our inner world." This runs counter to the classical notion that the left hemisphere is the "dominant" one and the right hemisphere the "minor" one, but it goes with the clinical finding that damage to the right hemisphere may have much stranger and profounder effects than the relatively straightforward effects of damage to the "dominant" hemisphere. Thus it is the integrity of the "minor" hemisphere, so-called, which Goldberg feels is crucial for the sense of self or identity—its integrity, and the integrity of the frontal lobes.

Another central theme of *The Executive Brain* relates to what Goldberg sees as the two radically different, but complementary, modes of cerebral organization. Classical neurology (and its precursor, phrenology) sees the brain as consisting of a multitude, a mosaic, of separate areas or systems or modules, each dedicated to a highly specific cognitive function, and all relatively isolated, with very limited interactions. Such an organization is evident in the more primitive parts of the brain, such as the thalamus (which consists of many discrete and separate nuclei) and the older parts of the cerebral cortex—thus the possibility of discrete, small lesions in the visual cortex producing equally discrete losses of color vision, movement vision, depth vision, etc. But such a system, Goldberg argues, would be rigid, not flexible, and have little capacity to deal with novelty or complexity, to adapt or learn. Such a system, he maintains, would be wholly inadequate to support identity or higher mental life.

Already in the 1960s, as a student, Goldberg was starting to envision a very different sort of organization in the newer and "higher" parts of the brain, the neocortex (which starts to develop in mammals and reaches its highest development in the human frontal lobes). A careful analysis of the effects of damage to the neocortex suggests that there are no longer discrete, isolated modules or domains here, but rather a gradual transition from one cognitive function to another, corresponding to a gradual, continuous trajectory along the cortical surface. Thus Goldberg's central concept is one of a cognitive continuum, a gradient. This radical idea enthralled the young Goldberg the more he thought of it: "I began to think of my gradients as the neuropsychological analogue of the Mendelev periodic table of elements." This gradiential theory was incubated and tested for twenty years, and was only written up by Goldberg in 1989, when he had gathered massive evidence to support it. The groundbreaking paper in which he launched his theory was largely ignored, despite the great explanatory power it promised.

When I wrote an essay in 1995 on prematurity in science [O. W. Sacks, "Scotoma: Forgetting and Neglect in Science," in Hidden Histories of Science, Ed. R. B. Silver (New York: New York Review of Books, 1996), 141–187.], I cited, among many other examples, the failure to comprehend or see the relevance of gradiential theory when it was published; Luria himself found it incomprehensible in 1969, when Goldberg first presented it to him. But there has been a great change, a paradigm shift (as Kuhn would say) in the last decade, partly connected with theories of global brain function such as Gerald Edelman's, partly with the development of neural nets as modelling systems, massively parallel computer systems, and the like, and the concept of cerebral gradients—Goldberg's vision as a student—is now much more widely accepted.

Modularity still exists, Goldberg emphasizes, as a persistent but archaic principle of cerebral organization, which was gradually supplanted or supplemented by a gradiential principle later in evolution. "If this is so," he remarks, "then an uncanny parallel exists between the evolution of the brain and the intellectual evolution of how we think about the brain. Both the evolution of the brain itself and the evolution of our theories about the brain have been characterized by a paradigmatic shift, from modular to interactive."

Goldberg wonders whether this paradigmatic shift may find parallels in political organization, with the breakup of large "macronational" states to smaller "microregional" states, a change which threatens anarchy unless a new supranational executive—the political equivalent of the frontal lobes—can arise and coordinate the new order of the world. He wonders, too, whether the replacement of the enormous but relatively few and isolated supercomputers of the 1970s by the hundreds of millions of personal computers which we have now, all potentially interacting, parallels the shift from modular to interactive, with search engines as the digital equivalent of frontal lobes.

The Executive Brain ends as it begins, on a personal and introspective note, with Goldberg's memory of how as a boy he read Spinoza in his father's library and loved Spinoza's calm equation of body and mind; and how this played a crucial part in directing him toward neuropsychology, and to avoiding that fatal splitting of body and mind, the dualism which Antonio Damasio calls "Descartes' error." Spinoza had no sense that the human mind, with its noble powers and aspirations, was in any way devalued or reduced by being dependent on the operations of a physical agency, the brain. One should rather, he said, admire the living body, for its wonderful and almost incomprehensible subtlety and complexity. It is only now, at the dawn of the 21st century, that we are beginning to get the full measure of this complexity, to see how nature and culture interact, and how brain and mind produce each other. There are a handful, a small handful, of remarkable books which address these central problems with great force—those of Gerald Edelman and Antonio Damasio at once come to mind—and to this select number, Elkhonon Goldberg's book *The Executive Brain* should surely be added.

Acknowledgments

I undertook the writing of this book, in a language still not entirely my own, with hesitation. By habit and temperament a prose terser than that expected of a semi-popular book comes more naturally to me. But I followed the proddings of several friends and went ahead, for two reasons. The better articulated reason was a growing realization that to make an impact, a writer sometimes needs to reach beyond the format of narrowly circulated scientific journals. The more elusive reason was a need to reconnect my Russian and American lives (at the time of this writing almost exactly equal in length) through a continuous personal intellectual narrative.

I owe a debt of gratitude to many people. To Oliver Sacks, a close friend of many years—the very proposition of writing a book for the general public would probably not have occurred to me without Oliver's example. To Dmitri Bougakov for technical editing, verifying facts and references, and helping design illustrations. To Laura Albritton, who helped edit the manuscript. To Fiona Stevens of Oxford University Press, who helped shepherd the book to publication. To Sergey Knyazev for his insightful discussion of the analogies between the brain and computers. To Vladimir and Kevin for giving me an opportunity to learn from their conditions. To those called Toby and Charlie as well as Lowell Handler and Shane Fistell for sharing their life stories and allowing me to describe them in this book. To Kevin's father for allowing me to write about his son. To Robert Iacono for sharing his experience with cingulotomy. To Peter Fitzgerald, Ida Bagus Made Adnyana, Kate Edgar, Wendy James,

Lewis Lerman, Jae Llewellyn-Kirby, Gus Norris, Martin Ozer, Peter Lang, Anne Veneziano, and Oxford's anonymous reviewers for valuable comments on the manuscript. To Brendon Connors, Dan Demetriad, Kamran Fallahpour, Evian Gordon, and Konstantin Pio-Ulsky for helping create some of the images used in the book. To my patients, friends, and acquaintances, who informed my work with their lives, tragedies, and triumphs and gave me the permission to write about them. To my students, who provided a captive audience in front of which I was able to rehearse pieces of the book. To the designers of the Psion palm-held computer, who enabled me to write the whole book out of my head in all kinds of improbable places. The book is dedicated to Alexandr Romanovich Luria, who referred to the frontal lobes as the "organ of civilization" and who had a greater impact on my career than I could remotely imagine while being his student.

New York, N.Y. E. G.

Contents

1. Introduction 1

2. An End and a Beginning: A Dedication 7

3. The Brain's Chief Executive: The Frontal Lobes at a Glance 21
The Many Faces of Leadership 21
The Executive Lobe 23

4. Architecture of the Brain: A Primer 27
The Microscopic View 27
The Macroscopic View 29
The Command Post and its Connections 35

5. The Orchestra's Front Row: The Cortex 37
Sounds and Players 37
Novelty, Routines, and Cerebral Hemispheres 40
Noah's Predicament and the Landscapes of the Brain 52
Module Madness 55
Cognitive Gradients and Cognitive Hierarchies 58
A Thing is a Thing 62
A Word to a Thing 64

6. The Conductor: A Closer Look at the Frontal Lobes 69
Novelty and the Frontal Lobes 69

Working Memory—or Working with Memory? 72
Freedom of Choice, Ambiguity, and the Frontal Lobes 77

7. Different Lobes for Different Folks: Decision-Making Styles and the Frontal Lobes 87
The Neuropsychology of Individual Differences 87
Male and Female Cognitive Styles 88
Frontal Lobes, Hemispheres, and Cognitive Styles 93
Cognitive Styles and Brain Wiring 96
Rebels in Small Proportion: Handedness and Novelty Seeking 99
Executive Talents: The *S* Factor and the Theory of Mind 104

8. When the Leader Is Wounded 113
The Fragile Frontal Lobes 113
Frontal Lobe Syndromes 116
Drive and Newtonian Bodies: A Dorsolateral Case Study 118
Plans and the "Memories of the Future" 123
Rigidity of Mind 129
Mind Blindspot: Anosognosia 135

9. Social Maturity, Morality, Law, and the Frontal Lobes 139
Orbitofrontal "Pseudopsychopathic" Syndrome and the Loss of Self-Control 139
Social Maturity and the Frontal Lobes 141
Biological Maturation and Social Maturity: A Historical Puzzle 143
Frontal Lobe Damage and Criminal Behavior 146
The Hapless Robber 150
Frontal Lobe Damage and the Public Blindspot 155

10. Fateful Disconnections 157
The Fallen Horseman: A Case Study 157
Schizophrenia: A Connection that Was Never Made 163
Head Trauma: A Broken Connection 167
Attention Deficit/Hyperactivity Disorder: A Fragile Connection 168

ADHD Conquered: How Toby from Down Under Reclaimed Himself 173
Jerky Tics and Ticky Jokes 180

11. "What Can You Do for Me?" 193
"Cognotropic" Drugs 193
Jogging the Brain 197
History of Cognitive Rehabilitation 202
Brain Plasticity and Cognitive Exercise 204
Cognitive Fitness: Beginning of a Trend 210
Beginnings of a Program 212

12. Frontal Lobes and the Leadership Paradox 215
Autonomy and Control in the Brain 215
Autonomy and Control in Society 219
Autonomy and Control in the Digital World 223

Epilogue 227

References and Notes 231

Index 247

1

Introduction

I began this book with a general audience in mind. But halfway through the project the professional in me prevailed over the popularizer, and the book is somewhat of a hybrid. At the risk of appealing to neither, I have tried to write a book that would appeal both to the general public and to the professional audience. Chapters 1, 2, 3, 9, 10, 11, 12 and the Epilogue are least technical and are of general interest; they should appeal both to the general reader and to professionals. Chapters 4, 5, 6, 7, and 8 are somewhat more technical but accessible to the general reader nonetheless. They deal with broad issues of cognitive neuroscience, of interest to scientists and clinicians as well as the general reader interested in the workings of the brain and the mind. The book does not represent an attempt at an encyclopedic, textbooklike account of the frontal lobes. Rather, it is an idiosyncratic account of my own understanding of several central issues of cognitive neuroscience and of the personal context that led me to write about it.

In this book I explore the one part of your brain that makes you who you are and defines your identity, that encapsulates your drives, your ambitions, your personality, your essence: the frontal lobes of the brain. If other parts of the brain are damaged, neurological illness can result in the loss of language, memory, perception, or movement. Yet the essence of the individual, the personality core, usually remains intact. All this changes when illness strikes at the frontal lobes. What is lost then is no longer an attribute of your mind. It *is* your mind, your core, your self. The frontal lobes are the most uniquely human of all the brain structures, and they play a critical role in the success or failure of any human endeavor.

"Descartes' error," to borrow the elegant phrase of Antonio Damasio,[1] consisted in believing that the mind has a life of its own independent of the body. Today a literate society no longer believes in the Cartesian dualism between body and mind, but we shed the vestiges of the old misconception in stages. Today few educated people, no matter how unschooled in neurobiology, doubt that language, movement, perception, memory all somehow reside in the brain. Yet ambition, drive, foresight, insight—those attributes that define one's personality and essence—are to this day viewed by many as, shall we say, "extracranial," as if they were attributes of our clothes and not our biology. These elusive human qualities are also controlled by the brain, and particularly by the frontal lobes. The prefrontal cortex is the focus of neuroscientific research today, yet it is largely unknown to non-scientists.

The frontal lobes perform the most advanced and complex functions in all of the brain, the so-called executive functions. They are linked to intentionality, purposefulness, and complex decision making. They reach significant development only in humans; arguably, they make us human. The entire human evolution has been termed "the age of the frontal lobes." My teacher Alexandr Luria called the frontal lobes "the organ of civilization."

This book is about leadership. The frontal lobes are to the brain what a conductor is to an orchestra, a general to an army, the chief executive officer to a corporation. They coordinate and lead other neural structures in concerted action. The frontal lobes are the brain's command post. We will examine how the leadership role evolved in various facets of human society—and in the brain.

This book is about motivation, drive, and vision. Motivation, drive, foresight, and clear vision of one's goals are central to success in any walk of life. You will discover how all these prerequisites of success are controlled by the frontal lobes. This book will also tell you about how even subtle damage to the frontal lobes produces apathy, inertia, and indifference.

This book is about self-awareness and awareness of others. Our ability to accomplish our goals depends on our ability to critically appraise our own actions and the actions of those around us. This ability rests with the frontal lobes. Damage to the frontal lobes produces debilitating blindness in judgement.

This book is about talent and success. We readily recognize literary talent, musical talent, athletic talent. But in a complex society such as ours a different talent comes to the fore, the leadership talent. Of all the forms of talent, the ability to lead, to compel other human beings to rally behind you, is the most mysterious and the most profound. In human history the leadership talent has had the greatest impact on the destinies of others and on personal success. This book highlights an intimate relationship between leadership and the frontal lobes. Of course, the converse of this is that poor frontal lobe function is especially devastating to an individual. Therefore, this book is also about failure.

This book is about creativity. Intelligence and creativity are inseparable yet not the same. Each of us has known people who are bright, intelligent, thoughtful—and barren. Creativity requires the ability to embrace novelty. We will examine the critical role of the frontal lobes in dealing with novelty.

This book is about men and women. Neuroscientists are only now beginning to study what people on the street have assumed all along, that men and women are different. Men and women approach things differently, they have different cognitive styles. We will examine how these differences in cognitive styles reflect the gender differences in the frontal lobes.

This book is about society and history. All complex systems have certain features in common, and by learning about one such a system we learn about the others. We will examine analogies between the evolution of the brain and the development of complex societal structures, and we will derive certain lessons about our own society.

This book is about social maturity and social responsibility. Frontal lobes define us as social beings. It is more than coincidence that the biological maturation of the frontal lobes takes place at the age that has been codified in virtually all developed cultures as the beginning of adulthood. But poor development of, or damage to, the frontal lobes may produce behavior devoid of social constraints and sense of responsibility. We will discuss how frontal lobe dysfunction may contribute to criminal behavior.

This book is about cognitive development and learning. Frontal lobes are critical for every successful learning process, for motivation and attention. Today we are increasingly aware of subtle disorders afflicting both children and adults—attention deficit disorder (ADD) and attention deficit hyperactivity disorder (ADHD).[2] This book describes how ADD and ADHD are caused by subtle dysfunction of the frontal lobes and the pathways connecting them to other parts of the brain.

This book is about aging. As we age, we are increasingly concerned about our mental astuteness. As popular concern about cognitive decline grows, everyone is talking about memory loss and no one speaks of the loss of executive functions. This book tells you how vulnerable the frontal lobes are in Alzheimer's disease and other dementias.

This book is about neurological and psychiatric illness. The frontal lobes are exceptionally fragile. Recent studies have shown that frontal lobe dysfunction is at the core of devastating disorders, such as schizophrenia and head trauma. Frontal lobes are also involved in Tourette's syndrome and obsessive-compulsive disorder.

This book is about enhancing your cognitive functions and protecting your mind against decline. Contemporary neuroscience is only now beginning to address these issues. Some of the latest ideas and approaches are reviewed here.

Above all, this book is about the *brain*, the mysterious organ that is part of us, that makes us who we are, that endows us with our powers and weighs us down with our weaknesses, the microcosm, the last frontier. In writing the book, I made no attempt to be dispassionately encyclopedic. I intended, rather, to present a distinctly personal, original, and at times provocative viewpoint on a number of topics in neuropsychology and cognitive neuroscience. Although many of these points were published earlier in scientific journals, they do not necessarily represent the prevailing opinion in the field, and many of them remain distinctly partisan, controversial, my own.

Finally, this book is about *people*: about my patients, my friends, and my teachers, who in various ways and on both sides of the iron curtain helped shape my interests and my career, thus making this book possible. The book is dedicated to Alexandr Romanovich Luria, the great neuropsychologist, whose legacy informed and shaped the field like nobody else's. As I referred to him elsewhere, he was, at various times, "my professor, my mentor, my friend, and my tyrant."[3] Our relationship was close and complex. In Chapter 2 I give a very personal account of one of the greatest psychologists of our time and of the extraordinarily difficult context in which he worked.

A socialite friend of mine remarked, succinctly and to the point: "Brain is great!" Among all the intellectual, quasi-intellectual, and pseudo-intellectual fads today, the popular interest in the brain reigns supreme. It is shared by an enlightened general public driven by genuine curiosity about the "science's last frontier"; by parents, eager for their children to succeed and dreading the prospect of failure; and by insatiable baby boomers, determined to remain in the driver's seat forever, but approaching the age when debilitating mental decline becomes a statistical possibility. To meet this unparalleled interest, scores of popular books have been written about memory, language, attention, emotion, cerebral hemispheres, and related subjects. Incredibly, though, one part of the brain has been completely ignored in this genre: the frontal lobes. This book has been written to fill the gap.

The educated public is becoming disabused of the blissful Cartesian delusion that the body is frail but the mind is forever. As we live longer, are better educated, and get ahead by our brain rather than brawn, we are increasingly interested in our minds and concerned about losing them.

Our self-centered society's preoccupation with illness has created a complex tangle of reality, neurosis, and guilt with doomsday overtones. Never too far from the center of our collective consciousness, this preoccupation usually focuses on one illness encapsulating all our fears, thus becoming, in the words of Susan Sontag,[4] a metaphor. It has been cancer, then acquired immunodeficiency syndrome (AIDS). As the shock value and novelty of the metaphor du jour wear off and familiarity breeds a (magical) sense of security, a new focus arises. During the 1990s, declared by the National Institutes of Health to be "the decade of the brain," dementia became, appropriately, the new focus. Since with age dementia strikes a significant proportion of the population, the concern is basically rational but, like most fads, takes on neurotic overtones.

As behooves a movement, the preoccupation with dementia has acquired its own metaphor, a metaphor within a metaphor, so to speak. The name of this metaphor is "memory." In the information society dominated by aging baby-boomers, there is a growing concern about forestalling cognitive decline and enhancing cognitive wellbeing. Memory clinics and memory-enhancing supplements proliferate. Major magazines are replete with features on memory. "Memory" has become the code name for the emerging mental fitness trend and the emerging preoccupation with losing one's mind, with dementia.

But cognition consists of many elements, memory being only one of them. Memory is one of many aspects of the mind central to our existence. Memory decline is only one of many ways in which the mind can be lost, just as Alzheimer's disease is but one of the several still incurable dementias and AIDS is but one of several as yet incurable lethal infectious diseases. Although undoubtedly fragile, memory is by no means the only, and possibly not even the most vulnerable aspect of the mind, and memory loss is by no means the only way in which the mind can be lost. People often complain of deteriorating "memory" for lack of a better or more accurate term, when what ails them, in fact, is the decline of an entirely different aspect of cognition.

As this book will show, no other cognitive loss comes close to the loss of executive functions in the degree of devastation that it visits on one's mind and one's self. As we learn more about brain diseases, we discover that the frontal lobes are particularly affected in dementia, schizophrenia, traumatic head injury, attention deficit disorder, and a host of other disorders. The executive functions are affected in dementias both frequently and early.

Any future efforts to enhance cognitive longevity through mind-enhancing "cognotropic" pharmacology, cognitive exercise, or any other means will have to focus on the executive functions of the frontal lobes. This book reviews the emerging scientific methods designed to protect and enhance the mind in general and the executive functions of the frontal lobes in particular.

Finally, we will draw broad analogies between the development of the brain and the development of other complex systems, such as digital computational devices and society. These analogies are based on the assumption that all complex systems have certain fundamental features in common and understanding one complex system helps us understand the others.

I believe that ideas are best understood when considered in the context in which they arise. Therefore, interwoven with the discussion of various topics of cognitive neuroscience are personal vignettes about my teachers, about my friends, about myself, and about the times in which we lived.

2

An End and a Beginning: A Dedication

Petty gripes aside, we live in a forgiving world, where the margin of error is usually quite generous. I have always suspected that even in the highest reaches of power, decision making is a pretty sloppy process. Once in a while, however, situations arise in the life of a human being, and a society, which allow no margin of error. These critical situations tax the decision maker's executive abilities to their utmost. At the age of 53, I can think of only one such a situation in my life. For me, at the time already a student of executive functions, the experience had the dual significance of a personal drama and a practical study in the workings of the frontal lobes—my own.

My mentor, Alexandr Romanovich Luria, and I were immersed in a conversation that we had had a dozen times before. We were strolling away from Luria's Moscow apartment, up Frunze Street and on toward the Old Arbat.[1] We were proceeding cautiously, because Luria had broken his leg and developed a limp, which slowed his usually brisk walking pace. It was an early spring afternoon, Moscow was thawing after a frigid winter, and the plaza was getting crowded. But Luria was so imposingly professorial in his heavy, almost floor-length navy cashmere coat with an astrakhan collar and a matching hat that the crowd gave way.

The year was 1972. The country had lived through Stalin's murderous years, through the war, through more of Stalin's murderous years, and through Khrushchev's aborted thaw. People were no longer executed for dissent; they were merely jailed. The overriding public mood was no longer bone-chilling terror, but damp, resigned, stagnant hopelessness and indifference, a societal stupor of sorts. My mentor was 70 and I was 25. I was approaching the end of my *aspirantura,* a postgraduate course usually leading to a faculty position. We were talking about my future.

As on many occasions before, Alexandr Romanovich was saying that it was time for me to join the party—*the* party, the Communist Party of the Soviet Union. A party member himself, Luria offered to nominate me and to arrange the second nomination from Alexey Nikolayevich Leontyev, also an illustrious psychologist and our dean at the University of Moscow, with whom I was on generally cordial terms. Party membership was the first rung of the Soviet elite, an obligatory steppingstone for any serious aspirations in life. It was understood that party membership was a sine qua non for any career advancement in the Soviet Union.

It was also understood that nominating me for party membership was a very generous gesture both for Luria and Leontyev. I was a Jew from Latvia, which was regarded as an untrustworthy province, and of "bourgeois" background. My father had spent five years in the Gulag as an "enemy of the people." I did not exactly adhere to the Soviet ideal. By vouching for me Luria and Leontyev, the two paramount figures in Soviet psychology, ran the risk of irritating the university's party organization for pushing "another Jew" into the rarefied strata of the Soviet academic elite. But they were willing to do it, which meant that they wanted me to stay on at the University of Moscow as a junior faculty member. The two of them had protected me in various situations before, and they were prepared to support me again.

Again and again, however, I told Alexandr Romanovich that I was not going to join the party. On a dozen occasions over the past few years, whenever Luria brought it up, I would sidestep the subject, turning it into a joke, saying that I was too young, too immature, not yet ready. I did not want an open clash and Luria did not force one. But this time he was speaking with finality. And this time I said that I was not going to join the party because *I did not want to.*

Alexandr Romanovich Luria was arguably the most important Soviet psychologist of his time. His multifaceted career included groundbreaking cross-cultural and developmental studies, mostly in collaboration with his mentor Lev Semyonovich Vygotsky, one of the greatest psychologists of the twentieth century. But it was his contribution to neuropsychology that earned him truly international acclaim. Universally regarded as a founding father of neuropsychology, he studied the neural basis of language, memory, and, of course, executive functions. Among his contemporaries, nobody contributed to the understanding of the complex relationship between the brain and cognition more than Luria, and he was revered on both sides of the Atlantic (Fig. 2.1).

Born in 1902 into the family of a prominent Jewish physician, he had lived through the cultural ferment of the beginning of the century, the volatile years of the Russian revolution, the civil war, Stalin's purges, World War II, a second round of Stalin's purges, and finally a relative thaw. He witnessed the names of his two closest friends and mentors, Lev Vygotsky and Nicholai Bernstein, besmirched and their life's work banned from existence by the state. At various points in his life he was on the verge of incarceration in Stalin's Gulag but, unlike many other Soviet intellectuals, was never actually imprisoned. His career was a peculiar blend of an intellectual odyssey driven by a genuine, natural unfolding of scientific inquiry and a survival course on the Soviet ideological minefield.

Coming from the westernmost edge of the Soviet empire, from the Baltic city of Riga, I grew up in a "European" environment. Unlike the families of my Moscow friends, my parents' generation did not grow up under the Soviets. I had some sense of "European" culture and "European" identity. Among my professors at the University of Moscow, Luria was one of the very few recognizably "European," and this was one of the things that drew me to him. He was a multilingual, multitalented man of the world, completely at home with Western civilization.

But he was also a Soviet man used to making compromises in order to survive. I suspected that in the deepest recesses of his being there was a visceral fear of brutal, physical repression. I had known other people like him, and it seemed that the latent fear was forever with them, even when the circumstances had changed and the fear was no longer based in reality, until they died. This fear was the glue of the Soviet regime, and I imagine the glue of any other repressive regime, until its collapse. This duality of inner intellectual freedom, even haughtiness, and everyday accommodation was rather

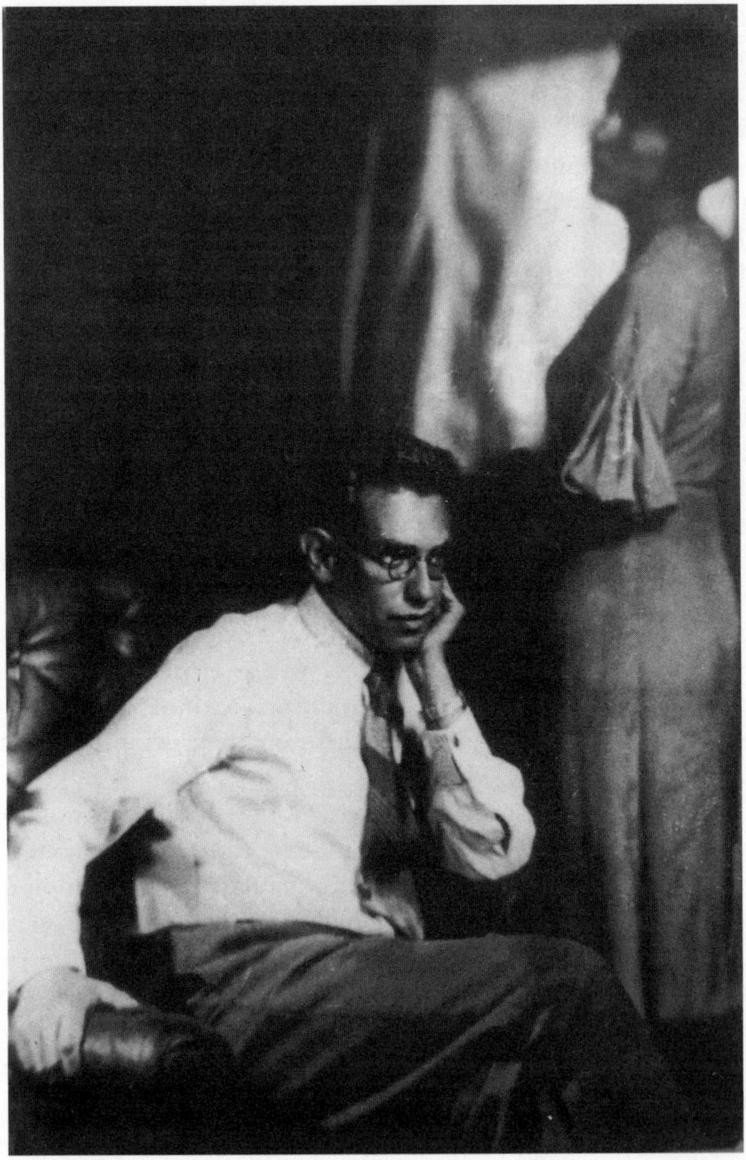

Figure 2.1. Alexandr Romanovich Luria and his wife Lana Pymenovna Luria, both in their early thirties. (Courtesy Dr. Lena Moskovich.)

common among the Soviet intelligentsia. I did not condemn Luria's party membership, but I did not respect it either, and it was a source of nagging ambivalence in my attitude toward him. I sort of pitied him for that, an odd feeling for a student to have toward a revered mentor.

My relations with Alexandr Romanovich and his wife Lana Pymenovna, herself a noted scientist-oncologist, were virtually familial. Warm and generous people, they had the habit of drawing their associates into their family life, inviting them to their Moscow apartment and country dacha, and taking them along to art exhibits. The youngest among Luria's immediate associates, I was often the object of their semiparental supervision, ranging from finding me a good dentist to reminders to shine my shoes. As is normal in life, we were occasionally at loggerheads in little things, but we were very close.

Now, as I stated point blank that I was not joining the party, Luria halted in the middle of the street. With a tinge of resignation but also a matter-of-fact finality, he said: "Then, Kolya (my old Russian nickname), there is nothing I can do for you." And that was that. This could have been devastating under a different set of circumstances, but that day I felt relief. Unbeknownst to Alexandr Romanovich or almost anyone else, I had already made up my mind to leave the Soviet Union. By making party membership a precondition for his continued patronage, he freed me from any obligation I felt toward him, which may have interfered with my decision. After this conversation, the last hesitation had been removed, and the question was no longer if, but how.

The decision to leave the country had developed gradually and my motives were complex. I lived under an oppressive regime. Yet my personal career had not been impeded up to that point. The state practiced tacit anti-Semitism; it was known that unwritten quotas existed at universities yet I studied at the best university in the land. It was known that generally the Jews were not welcome into the highest strata of the Soviet society yet I did not experience anti-Semitism directed at me personally. Most of my closest friends were Russian, and in my immediate social circle the issue of ethnicity simply did not arise. I was surrounded with successful Jews of my parents' generation, which meant that a career was possible in the Soviet Union despite the tacit restrictions. Religious practices were curtailed and impeded, but I grew up in a secular family and this was not an issue of personal concern.

Most of my friends understood that we lived in a society that was neither free nor affluent. Despite the Soviet grandstanding, there was a national sense of inferiority and a sense that the rest of the world was more vibrant, richer in opportunities. We were cut off from that world, the iron curtain a palpable reality, and the larger world beckoned. Having grown up in the Westernized Riga, I had no fear of that world.

Political indoctrination began in the Soviet Union practically from the nursery. But my family was a little enclave of passive dissent and I began to receive a healthy antidote against official propaganda very early in life. My father was sent to a labor camp when I was a year old. In a grim joke circulating around the country in those days, two inmates were chatting in a labor camp. "How much time did you get?" "Twenty years" "What did you do?" "I burned down a collective farm. And what did you do?" "Nothing" "How much time did you get?" "Fifteen years" "Rubbish. For nothing you get only ten."

My father was sentenced to ten years in the Gulag in western Siberia. He was sentenced as part of what I called "sociocide," a systematic extermination of whole social groups: the intelligentsia, the foreign-educated, the former affluent class. A mere membership in one of these groups marked you for persecution. My father was sent to a labor camp, and in the hallway of our apartment my mother kept two packed small suitcases, one for herself and one for me. Separate labor camps existed for the "wives of the enemies of the people," and special orphanages existed for the "children of the enemies of the people." Suitcases were packed and ready in many apartments across the land. The plainclothes agents of the state used to drive up in unmarked black cars (*voronki,* Russian for "little crows") without warning in the middle of the night, ring the doorbell, and give their victims 15 minutes to get ready, before taking them away for 5, 10, 20 years, or for good. One had to be prepared.

I grew up knowing that my father was far away, but not knowing where exactly. The address on his letters was just a "post office box," and as a child I kept wondering why my father had chosen to live in a box, far away. When Stalin's death was announced in April 1953, somber music was played across the city through loudspeakers. People were weeping on the streets. My mother rushed to the apartment pulling me along, unable to contain her joy and afraid to reveal it in public. My mother had always been politically vocal, to the point of recklessness. It was dangerous to confide even in one's own children, since they were encouraged to report on their parents—and some did. One of them, a boy by the name of Pavlik Morozov, had become a national hero.

Within months, many prisoners of the Gulag were released ahead of time, my father among them. I recall my mother falling into the embrace of a skeleton-thin stranger on the train station platform in Riga. I was six years of age and had no memories of my father. Only then did I find out that the "box" was a labor camp, and what this meant. That was my first insight into the true nature of the state we lived in. Many years later my mother recalled that I had thrown a fit of rage that frightened her by its intensity, screaming "So this is what the Soviet Union is really all about!"

Life soon settled into normalcy. As I was growing up, I had no illusions about the state I lived in and had no attachment to it in a patriotic sense. Far from it, by a certain age I developed a reasonably well-articulated sense that my whole Soviet existence was a regrettable accident of birth. Yet on a day-to-day level I felt comfortable and often happy, and I "blended in." I was accepted by the University of Moscow and was on my way to joining the academic elite. But gradually the realization grew that there was no future in the Soviet Union, just as there was no future for the Soviet Union.

And now I was standing in the middle of Arbat, knowing that the last source of hesitation had been removed. An existential decision now awaited an executive solution. An attempt to leave the country required an intricate plan, and there was no guarantee of success. To get out, I had to outsmart the Soviet state. I knew that my frontal lobes were going to be heavily taxed during the months to come.

The "workers' paradise" was designed like a mousetrap. It was easier to get in than out. Soviet citizens could not leave the country at will, even temporarily. Permission to go abroad as a tourist or in an official capacity already implied an elite status. A whole family was almost never allowed to travel together; a hostage was always kept to prevent defection. Emigrating permanently was even more difficult. Until the early seventies it was virtually unheard of. Then, as the consequence of détente and under the pressure from the United States Congress, limited emigration was allowed for Jews to go to Israel. By restricting emigration in this way, the authorities hoped that the precedent could be contained. In reality, however, once they were out of the country Jews were free to go where they chose. Many, myself included, chose the United States. This produced an ironic moment in the history of Russia, when being Jewish suddenly became an asset. I was a member of that all-of-a-sudden "privileged" minority. In that unique set of circumstances, my Jewishness provided a vehicle, more than an impetus, to attempt to get out. As is often the case in life, the relationship between a desire and an opportunity was a bit circular.

But there were many hurdles to jump. The Soviet state was brutally pragmatic. The greater the perceived value of the individual, the more difficult it was to get permission to leave the country. For the graduates of elite universities the chances approached zero. As a graduate of the Moscow State University, the Harvard of the East, I was a valued property of the state. People like me were not ordinarily allowed to emigrate. The slave-owning analogy extended further. Even if permission was granted in principle, the state exacted a ransom, which was determined based on a person's educational level. My ransom would be particularly exorbitant.

My doctoral dissertation had been written and bound, and the oral defense was scheduled in a few months. It was clear that I could not apply for an exit visa while still at the University of Moscow. Anyone applying for an exit visa was made an instant persona non grata. Nobody would allow me to defend my dissertation under these circumstances. I would be immediately expelled from the university.

Delaying my application until after my defense seemed like a logical thing to do. But as I was beginning to plot my escape, it became clear that an advanced degree would jeopardize my chances. Reluctantly, I was reaching the conclusion that I would have to somehow sabotage my own defense. As the frontal lobe functions go, this was an extreme case of inhibiting an urge for immediate gratification. I had to sacrifice something that I had striven for for several years and that would have been mine, with an assured outcome, in a few months' time. The delayed gratification was the prospect of getting out of the country. In the hierarchy of goals (prioritizing one's objectives, another frontal lobe function), this was a higher goal.

The strategy was not without risk. By not receiving my doctorate, I was merely enhancing my chance of success but by no means assuring it. The equation was too murky to compute the gain in probabilities with any degree of precision. Whatever it was, the probability remained high that I would not be allowed to leave. In situations like this, people remained in a lifelong limbo. Denied the request to leave the country, they were also denied the opportunity to reenter the mainstream of the Soviet society. They were fired from their positions and became lifelong pariahs, condemned to menial jobs on the fringes of society. But this is precisely why the doctorate no longer mattered. Refused the right to leave, I would be driving a taxi for a living with or without my doctorate.

And then there was another reason not to defend the dissertation: protecting my friends. My professors would be held responsible by the authorities for the "lack of political vigilance," for nurturing a future "traitor to the motherland." Bizarre as this vernacular sounded, it was actually used in the official political discourse in the Soviet Union. As my mentor, Alexandr Romanovich would be particularly affected. This had to be avoided.

Gradually, a plan took shape in my head. I would somehow avoid defending my dissertation. Then I would disappear from the University of Moscow as inconspicuously as possible and leave Moscow altogether. I would go to my native city of Riga and get the lowliest job possible. Then, after several months, or a year, I would apply for the exit visa. Then it would be out of my hands.

The exact timing of my application would have to depend on things not under my control. Détente was gathering steam. Henry Kissinger was in and out of the country. There were intimations in the press of an imminent visit by President Nixon. In those situations the Soviets tended to put on their liberal face. I was determined to painstakingly time my application to coincide with these events as precisely as possible. As I was thinking through the details of my plan, I had a strange sense of depersonalization, as if I was going through the plot of a novel about someone else's life. But this was to be my story, and it was self-inflicted.

I was trying to cover my tracks. Not that I believed that at the critical moment of decision the authorities would be ignorant of my past. You could not cover your tracks in the Soviet Union. Wherever you moved, you had to register with the local police. An internal file followed every Soviet citizen with every movement around the country. But I was counting on the indifferent and fundamentally brainless nature of the Soviet bureaucracy. By the 1970s, there were very few zealots left within the system. Things were done by the book. The book said that graduates of the University of Moscow and the like were valuable and should not be allowed to leave. The book also said that street-sweepers, cab drivers, and grocery clerks were dispensable and could be let go in the name of the lip service to détente. But the book said nothing about graduates of the University of Moscow turned street-sweepers. My gamble was that the authorities, in their mechanical ways, would not ruminate over my file.

There was another element in my calculations. In a tacit way, I was communicating to the authorities that I was not afraid of them. By relinquishing voluntarily the prestige and promise of my university position and assuming a menial job, I was, in a way, preempting them. I was visiting upon myself of my own accord everything they would have done to me had I applied for the exit visa while still at the University of Moscow. By robbing them of the means of repercussion, I robbed them of their control over me. Jailing me was the only thing left to them. Not being an active dissident, I did not think it likely. The less fear I showed, the more effort they knew it would take to intimidate me into retreat from my plan. With the détente in the air and their eagerness to look "civil," they were likely to conclude that keeping me was not worth the effort. But there was no guarantee.

My first impulse was to sit down with Alexandr Romanovich and reveal my plan to him. But there were two compelling reasons not to do so. Although I was doing all I could to distance myself from him, and thus minimize any possible repercussions of my actions for him, I could not be certain of his reaction. Whatever his true beliefs were, publicly he had always been a loyal, sometimes eagerly loyal, Soviet citizen. Was it only a patina, which he was careful not to drop? Did he truly believe what he said? I suspected that it was something in between, that a constant conscious dissonance between what you said and what you felt was too painful to endure. In many years of our close association, I was never able to have a candid political discussion with Alexandr Romanovich. Whenever I tried to draw him out, his response was a strident, almost frenzied "party line." The closest Luria had ever come to revealing his deeply buried discontent was through an occasional oblique muttering "Vremena slozhnye, durakov mnogo" ("These are complex times, many fools around"). What was first adopted as protective mimicry in time became a form of "autohypnosis."

Ironically, the term "autohypnosis" was proposed in 1990, half-jokingly, by none other than Luria's own daughter Lena over dinner at Nirvana, an Indian restaurant overlooking New York's Central Park. We were talking about her parents, both long deceased, and about other people of their generation. Like myself, Lena was fascinated by political autohypnosis as a psychological defense mechanism under tyranny. Luria's wife Lana Pymenovna was considerably less given to autohypnosis, and over the years we had had many candid conversations on forbidden subjects.

With this background, there was no guarantee that Luria would not report my intentions to the university authorities. According to the rules governing the system, this was actually expected of him, and ignoring the rule would be perceived as a serious transgression by a Soviet professor and party member in good standing. Informed about my plans, the university would get rid of me immediately as a potential source of embarrassment. I would find myself in an impossible limbo even before applying for the visa. That was particularly risky. Expelled from the university as "politically unsound," I would find it extremely difficult to get a job—any kind of job. Within the parameters of the Soviet mousetrap-state, this was a very dangerous place to be. A law on the books allowed the state to arrest and jail "parasites," people without employment. This rarely enforced law was invoked when the authorities wanted to "get" someone—particularly the "politically unsound" trying to leave the country. For the sake of my plan, and my teacher's soul, I could only hope that he would not turn me in, but there was no guarantee.

And then there was another, less self-centered reason not to confide in Alexandr Romanovich. Simply put, I was afraid that the shock of the news about my plans would trigger a heart attack right then and there. He did have a bad heart, and the visceral fear of the state could lead to an emotional reaction disproportionate to the reality of the situation. No matter how you looked at it, Alexandr Romanovich was better off not knowing about my intentions. Only a few people knew about my plans. They were all trusted friends, despite their very different origins and persuasions.

And so I decided to resort to a "white lie." Canceling an already scheduled oral defense was unheard of. I invented a story about a medical emergency in the family and the pressing need to get a job right away. My manifest plan was to move back to Riga, get a job, support my family until the "crisis" was over, and then come back to defend—in half a year or a year, with any luck. Luria was disturbed by the story, but through a tour de force I prevailed. I was able to disengage myself from the university without revealing, and thus jeopardizing, my plans.

I arrived in Riga and began to look for a job. This turned out to be very difficult, since I was obviously overqualified for the jobs I was applying for. Finally, I was hired as a hospital orderly at a downtown city hospital—the lowest on the totem pole. I was assigned to the emergency intensive care unit. The patients—car accidents, overdoses, stab wounds, rapes—gave me a new perspective on the city of my birth.

The patients were brought in by ambulance in the middle of the night. I reported for work at six in the morning, by which time some of them had passed away. Identifying the dead on the filthy beds and counting them was my first order of the day. Six or seven was about average. My duty was to deliver the cadavers to the morgue. I carried them manually on a shaky stretcher with my "partner," Maria.

Maria was a toothless, perpetually drunk woman of 40 going on 65. Her command of Russian profanities was awesome. I was, in those days, pretty foul-mouthed myself, yet I was humbled by her virtuosity. Every morning on arrival she checked out the medical autoclaves for ethanol used to sterilize medical instruments. This was her breakfast. By seven in the morning, when we were ready to load our cadavers, she was so drunk she could barely walk. She stumbled, tripped, and occasionally fell. Then I was stuck with two cadavers, a real one and a virtual one.

The rest of my activities were trivial by comparison: carrying bottles with medications, mopping floors, transferring patients—all the usual tasks orderlies do all over the world. It was a surreal experience. But after months of extreme cognitive exertion associated with critical decision making (this must have been the first time in my life when I discovered such a thing as cognitive exertion), there was calm, a hiatus, a semblance of stability, however fragile and bizarre. For the next few months, until I applied for my visa, there were no critical decisions to make. And when I applied, I would not be fired. Not from this job! I was resting my frontal lobes.

In due time I applied for my exit visa, and a few months later I was summoned to receive the response. It was favorable. I was free to go. The uniformed woman who gave me the news had my file in front of her. She browsed through it and exclaimed with incredulity: "They are letting you go with a background like this!" I just shrugged my shoulders. There was no indignation in her voice, just bemusement. It was not her decision and she did not care. There were few zealots left within the system. As I was walking down the street, I again had a sense of depersonalization, as if this was not happening to me but to someone I was watching from outside.

I flew to Moscow to say goodbyes. Like hundreds of times before, we were sitting together around the massive antique desk with brass lion heads in Luria's study. Two years had passed since our walk on the old Arbat. We, Alexandr Romanovich and I, talked for many hours, six, seven, or more. Lana Pymenovna was serving tea and joining us intermittently. Luria was not offended by my white lie. He sounded relieved to have been left out of the whole affair. Finally he said: "I don't approve of *what* you are doing, but I thank you for *how* you have done it." It was understood that I could never contact him from abroad, I was now persona non grata. This was to be our last conversation. Alexandr Romanovich died three years later.

And I came to the United States and started from the beginning. The intellectual and stylistic continuity linking a pupil to his master was broken and I found myself in my new homeland essentially on my own. This made things harder in the beginning, yet in retrospect more gratifying. But the continuity was also preserved through the numerous and enduring threads of my teacher's influences, which to this day permeate my career in ways both obvious and subtle. Exactly 27 years have passed since that uneasy farewell. My interest in the frontal lobes was seeded by Alexandr Romanovich and has remained among the most persistent themes of my career. And so this book is written in memory of Alexandr Romanovich Luria, the man who influenced my life in definitive ways, and of the complex times in which his career ended and mine began.

3

The Brain's Chief Executive: The Frontal Lobes at a Glance

The Many Faces of Leadership

They arrive at work in limousines with smoked glass windows; they ride to the top floors of the corporate headquarters in private elevators; their salaries are beyond the average person's imagination. An informal survey suggests that they are, on average, a few inches taller than the rest of us. Cloaked in mystique and regarded with awe, they are the chief executive officers—CEOs—of America.

Up the street from the soaring midtown Manhattan corporate headquarters, at Carnegie Hall, a disheveled conductor rehearses his orchestra. A few blocks south, off Broadway, an exasperated stage director tries to get actors to grasp his interpretation of a famous play. They would seem to have little in common with the corporate baron, but they perform similar functions. To a naive observer, the CEO does not manufacture the company's product, just as the conductor does not make music, and the director does not act. Yet they direct the actions of those who manufacture the product, play the music, or perform on the stage. Without them there would be no product, no concert, no show.

The role of a leader sending others into action, instead of acting himself, evolved in society relatively late. The history of early music makes no mention of the conductor, and there is no mention of a director in the Greek theater. Early warfare was a clash of two hordes, each man fighting his own fight; the general came millennia later. And it was fairly recently in the history of warfare that the top military commander no longer inspired the troops with his personal frontline courage but guided the battle from the rear.[1]

The function of leadership acquires a distinct status and becomes separate only when the size and complexity of the organization (or the organism) crosses a certain threshold. Once the function of leadership has crystallized into a specialized role, the wisdom of leadership is to maintain a delicate, dynamic balance between the autonomy of, and control over, the organism's parts. A wise leader knows when to step in and impose his will and when to step back and let his lieutenants display their own initiative.

The leader's role is elusive but critical. Let the leader lapse, however briefly, and disaster strikes. An orchestra will descend into cacophony, corporate decision making will grind to a halt, and a great army will falter. In fact, some historians attribute the decisive defeat of Napoleon's Great Army at Waterloo to the emperor's flagging leadership due to a painful exacerbation of chronic illness.[2]

The leader's role is critical but elusive. I recall wondering, as a little boy, why the orchestra required that funny man on the podium waving his hands, since he did not contribute anything audible to the music created before me. And I recall my friend's three-year-old son describing his father's job as "sitting in the office and sharpening pencils" (his father was the chairman of a large department at a major university).

Likewise, early neurology texts contained elaborate descriptions of the roles played by other parts of the brain but gave the frontal lobes barely a footnote. The implication was that the frontal lobes were there mostly for ornamental purposes. It took neuroscientists many years to even begin to appreciate the importance of the frontal lobes for cognition. But when this finally happened, a picture of particular complexity and elegance emerged. We will begin to examine it now.

The Executive Lobe

The human brain is the most complex natural system in the known universe; its complexity rivals, and probably exceeds, the complexity of the most intricate social and economic structures. It is science's new frontier. The 1990s were declared by the National Institutes of Health the decade of the brain. Just as the first half of the twentieth century was the age of physics, and the second half of the twentieth century was the age of biology, so the beginning of the twenty-first century is the age of brain–mind science.

Like a large corporation, a large orchestra, or a large army, the brain consists of distinct components serving distinct functions. And like these large-scale human organizations, the brain has its CEO, its conductor, its general: the frontal lobes. To be precise, this role is vested in but one part of the frontal lobes, the prefrontal cortex. It is a common shorthand, however, to use the term "frontal lobes."

Like the exalted leadership roles in human society, the frontal lobes were late in coming. In evolution their development began to accelerate only with the great apes. As the seat of intentionality, foresight, and planning, the frontal lobes are the most uniquely "human" of all the components of the human brain. In 1928 the neurologist Tilney suggested that entire human evolution should be considered the "age of the frontal lobe."[3]

Like the functions of a CEO, the functions of the frontal lobes defy a soundbite definition. They are not invested with any single, ready-to-label function. A patient with frontal lobe disease will retain the ability to move around, use language, recognize objects, and even memorize information. Yet like a leaderless army, cognition disintegrates and ultimately collapses with the loss of the frontal lobes. In my native Russian language, there is an expression "bez tsarya v golovye," "a head without the czar inside." This expression could have been invented to describe the effects of frontal lobe damage on behavior.

As if the royal connection was not enough, the frontal lobes have been invested also with divine aura. In his remarkable cultural–neuropsychological essay Julian Jaynes advances the idea that internally generated executive commands were mistaken by primitive man for externally originated voices of the gods.[4] Thus, by implication, the advent of executive functions at early stages of human civilization may have been responsible for the molding of religious beliefs.

Art historians have noted a curious detail in *The Creation of Adam*, Michelangelo's great fresco on the ceiling of the Sistine Chapel. God's mantle has the distinct shape of the outline of the brain, his feet rest on the brain stem, and his head is framed by the frontal lobe. God's finger, pointed toward Adam and making him human, projects from the prefrontal cortex. In the words of Julius Meier-Graefe, "There is more genius in the finger of God, calling Adam to life, than in the whole work of any of Michelangelo's forerunners."[5] No one knows whether the allegory was intended by Michelangelo, or whether the image is coincidental; it may well be the latter. But a more powerful symbol of the frontal lobes' profound humanizing effect can hardly be imagined. The frontal lobes are truly "the organ of civilization."

Because the frontal lobes are not linked to any single, easily defined function, early theories of brain organization denied them any role of consequence. In fact, the frontal lobes used to be known as "the silent lobes." Over the last decades, however, the frontal lobes have become the focus of intense scientific investigation. Still, our efforts to understand the functions of the frontal lobes, and particularly the prefrontal cortex, are very much a work in progress and, for lack of more precise concepts, we often lapse into poetic metaphor. The prefrontal cortex plays the central role in forming goals and objectives and then in devising plans of action required to attain these goals. It selects the cognitive skills required to implement the plans, coordinates these skills, and applies them in a correct order. Finally, the prefrontal cortex is responsible for evaluating our actions as success or failure relative to our intentions.

Human cognition is forward-looking, proactive rather than reactive. It is driven by goals, plans, aspirations, ambitions, and dreams, all of which pertain to the future and not to the past. These cognitive powers depend on the frontal lobes and evolve with them. In a broad sense, the frontal lobes are the organism's mechanism of liberating itself from the past and projecting into the future. The frontal lobes endow the organism with the ability to create neural models of things as a prerequisite for making things happen, models of something that does not yet exist but which you want to bring into existence.

To conjure up an internal representation of the future, the brain must have an ability to take certain elements of prior experiences and reconfigure them in a way that in its totality does not correspond to any actual past experience. To accomplish this, the organism must go beyond the mere ability to *form* internal representations, the models of the world outside. It must acquire the ability to *manipulate* and *transform* these models. As a friend of mine, a gifted mathematician, has said, the organism must go beyond the ability to see the world *through* mental representations; it must acquire the ability to work *with* mental representations. One of the fundamental distinguishing features of human cognition, systematic tool making, may be said to depend on this ability, since a tool does not exist in a ready-made form in the natural environment and has to be conjured in order to be made. To go even further, the development of the neural machinery capable of creating and holding images of the future, the frontal lobes, may be seen as a necessary prerequisite for tool making, and thus for the ascent of man and the launching of human civilization as it is frequently defined.

Moreover, the generative power of language to create new constructs may depend on this ability as well. The ability to manipulate and recombine internal representations critically depends on the prefrontal cortex, and the emergence of this ability parallels the evolution of the frontal lobes. If there is such a thing as "the language instinct,"[6] it may be related to the emergence, late in evolution, of the functional properties of the frontal lobes.

Therefore, the roughly contemporaneous development of executive functions and language was adaptively highly fortuitous. Language provided the means for building models and the executive functions the means of manipulating them and conducting operations on the models. To parlay this into the language of biology, the advent of the frontal lobes was necessary to make use of the generative capability inherent in language. For the believers in drastic discontinuities as a major factor in evolution, the confluence between the development of language and executive functions may have been the definitive force behind the quantum leap that was the advent of man.

Of all the mental processes, goal formation is the most actor-centered activity. Goal formation is about "I need" and not about "it is." So the emergence of the ability to formulate goals must have been inexorably linked to the emergence of the mental representation of "self." It should come as no surprise that the emergence of self-consciousness is also intricately linked to the evolution of the frontal lobes.

All these functions can be thought of as metacognitive rather than cognitive, since they do not refer to any particular mental skill but provide an overarching organization for all of them. For this reason some authors refer to the functions of the frontal lobes as "executive functions," by analogy with the corporate CEO. I find the analogy with the orchestra conductor even more revealing. But to fully appreciate the functions and the responsibilities of the conductor, we first need to learn more about the orchestra.

4

Architecture of the Brain: A Primer

The Microscopic View

The brain consists of hundreds of billions of cells (*neurons* and *glial cells*), intricately interconnected by pathways (*dendrites* and *axons*). Several types of neurons and glial cells exist. Some of the pathways between neurons are local, branching within their immediate "neighborhoods." But others are long, interconnecting distant neural structures. These long pathways are covered with white fatty tissue, *myelin,* which facilitates the passage of the electric signals generated within the neurons (*action potentials*). The neurons and short local connections together comprise the *gray matter,* and the long myelinated pathways comprise the *white matter.* Every neuron is interconnected with a myriad of other neurons, resulting in intricate patterns of interactions. Thus a network of mind-boggling complexity is constructed of relatively simple elements.

The principle of achieving great complexity through multiple permutations of simple elements appears to be universal and is implemented in nature (and culture) in a variety of ways. Think, for instance, of language, where thousands of words, sentences, and narratives are constructed out of a few dozen letters; or think of the genetic code, where a virtually infinite number of variants can be achieved through the combination of a finite number of genes.

Although the signal generated within a neuron is electric, the communication between the neurons takes a chemical form. Intertwined and interwoven with the structural complexity described above are the brain's multiple biochemical systems. The biochemical substances, called *neurotransmitters* and *neuromodulators*, allow communication between neurons. An electric signal (*action potential*) is generated within the body of the neuron and travels along the axon until it reaches the terminal, the point of contact with a dendrite, a pathway leading to another neuron. At the point of contact there is a gap called the *synapse.* The arrival of the action potential releases small quantities of chemical substances (neurotransmitters), which travel across the synapse like rafts across a river and attach themselves to *receptors*, highly specialized molecules on the other side of the gap. This accomplished, the neurotransmitters are broken down in the synapse with the help of specialized enzymes. Meanwhile, the activation of postsynaptic receptors results in another electric event, a *postsynaptic potential.* A number of postsynaptic potentials occurring together result in another action potential, and the process is iterated thousands of thousands of times along both parallel and sequential pathways. This allows coding information of stupendous complexity.

We are constantly learning about new types of neurotransmitters. To date, several dozens of them have been discovered: glutamate, gamma-aminobutyric acid (GABA), serotonin, acetylcholine, norepinephrine, and dopamine, to name a few. Some neurotransmitters, like glutamate or GABA, are found virtually everywhere in the brain. Other neurotransmitters, like dopamine, are restricted to certain parts of the brain. Each neurotransmitter can bind to several receptor types, some of which are ubiquitous and others region-specific.

The brain can be thought of as the coupling of two highly complex organizations, structural and chemical. This coupling leads to an exponential increase in the system's overall complexity. This, in turn, is further increased by the ubiquitous feedback loops with the activity of the signal source being modified by its target, both local and global, both structural and biochemical. As a result, the brain can produce a virtually infinite array of different activation patterns, corresponding to the virtually infinite states of the outside world. The neuron represents a microscopic unit of the brain, and the pattern of connectivity between neurons represents the microscopic organization of the brain.

When the organism is exposed to a new pattern of signals from the outside world, the strengths of synaptic contacts (the ease of signal passage between neurons) and local biochemical and electric properties gradually change in complex distributed constellations. This represents learning, as we understand it today.[1]

The Macroscopic View

Neurons are grouped into cohesive structures, *nuclei* and *regions*. Each structure consists of millions of neurons. The nuclei and regions represent the macroscopic units of the brain, and the pattern of connectivity between them represents the macroscopic organization of the brain. The brain is a highly interconnected system, and the architecture of the major connections between its nuclei and regions provides a useful aerial view of the whole system.

For heuristic purposes, I resort to the metaphor of a tree. A tree has a trunk and branches. Branches divide into limbs. At the end of the limbs sits fruit. In a way, the brain is organized in a similar manner. One can think of the brain as an "arousal and activation tree." Its trunk is in charge of the general physiological arousal and activation necessary for the function of various brain structures, the fruit. This is the brain's anatomical pivot, the *brain stem*. Massive damage to the brain stem disrupts consciousness and may lead to coma.

Contained within the compact brain stem core are numerous nuclei, which give rise to an intricate system of pathways. In many instances the nuclei and their projections are biochemically specific, linked to a particular neurotransmitter; in other instances they are biochemically complex, involving several neurotransmitters. These are the branches and limbs of the "arousal tree." Each branch contains projections to a distinct part of the brain, ensuring its activation. A few decades ago it was common to refer to these branches collectively as the ascending reticular activating system (ARAS).[2] Today it is increasingly possible to identify its distinct neuroanatomical and biochemical components and to study these components separately. Damage to any given branch will not disrupt consciousness in a global sense, but will interfere with specific brain function. Each branch of the arousal tree projects into distinct components of the brain, each with its own set of functions.

A number of subcortical structures exist in the brain. In evolution, subcortical structures developed before the cortex, and for millions of years they guided the complex behaviors of various organisms. In contemporary living reptiles, and even birds, neocortex is only minimally represented.[3] In a phylogenetically ancient, acortical brain two sets of structures could be identified: the *thalamus* and the *basal ganglia.* Early in evolution the central nervous system divided into two lateral halves. Therefore, each of the brain structures described here consists of a pair of twin halves: left and right.

Despite a certain functional overlap, the thalamus and the basal ganglia were invested with distinctly different functions. In the ancient, precortical brain the thalamus was mostly in charge of receiving and processing information from the external world, and the basal ganglia were in charge of motor behavior and action. Thus the distinction between perception and action seems to have been fundamental in the brain's architecture from early on. The arousal tree divides into two major branches, one projecting separately into the subcortical machinery of perception (the *dorsal branch*), the other one of action (the *ventral branch*).

Although often treated as a single structure, the thalamus is, in fact, a collection of many nuclei. Some of them are in charge of processing distinct types of sensory information: visual, auditory, tactile, and the like. Other thalamic nuclei are in charge of integrating various types of sensory information. A complex hierarchy of input integration is present in the thalamus. The dorsomedial thalamic nucleus is at the summit of this hierarchy, and it is closely interconnected with the prefrontal cortex. Other thalamic nuclei, found around the midline, are nonspecific, in charge of various forms of activation.[4]

Closely linked to the thalamus is a structure called the *hypothalamus.* While the thalamus monitors the world outside, the hypothalamus monitors the organism's internal states and helps maintain them within the adaptive, homeostatic parameters. The hypothalamus is also a collection of distinct nuclei, each related to a distinct aspect of homeostasis: food intake, liquid intake, body temperature, and so on. Together, the thalamus and the hypothalamus are referred as the *diencephalon.*[5]

The basal ganglia include the caudate nuclei, the putamen, and globus pallidus. In the precortical brain these structures were central to the initiation of actions and control over movements. In the evolved mammalian brain the basal ganglia are under particularly close control of the frontal lobes and work in collaboration with them. In fact, the collaboration is so close that I tend to think of the caudate nuclei as part of the "greater frontal lobes."

A structure called the *amygdala* is also regarded as one of the basal ganglia, but it serves a somewhat different function. The amygdala regulates those interactions of the organism with the external world which are critical to the survival of the specimen and the species: decisions to attack or to escape, to copulate or not, to ingest or not. It provides rapid, precognitive, affective assessment of the situation in terms of its survival value.[6]

The *cerebellum* is a large structure attached to the back (or as a neuroanatomist would say, to the dorsal aspect) of the brain stem. Its anatomy parallels in miniature the anatomy of the whole brain: a pivot called the vermis and two cerebellar hemispheres. The cerebellum is important in movements, particularly in coordinating fine movements with sensory information. But recent studies have also shown that the cerebellum is closely linked to the frontal cortex and participates in complex planning.[7]

Relatively late in the evolution of the brain, the cortex began to emerge, first archicortex, then paleocortex.[8] They include the hippocampus and the cingulate cortex. The *hippocampus*, the "seahorse," is composed of two long structures hugging the inside of the temporal lobes (or as a neuroanatomist would say, on their mesial aspects). The hippocampus plays a critical role in memory. Some scientists believe that it is dedicated particularly to spatial learning.[9] I think that this is a narrow view prompted by animal experiments, where spatial learning is the only possible paradigm to study memory. In humans, the hippocampus is also implicated in other forms of memory, such as verbal memory.[10]

The *cingulate cortex* hugs the inner surface of the hemispheres overlying the corpus callosum. Its function is not entirely clear, but it has been implicated in emotions. Together with the amygdala and hippocampi, the cingulate cortex comprises the so-called limbic system,[11] a somewhat outdated construct implying a functional unity among these structures, whose heuristic value has been increasingly challenged. The anterior cingulate cortex, presumed to deal with uncertainty, is closely linked to the prefrontal cortex.[12] In a sense, it is also part of the greater frontal lobes.

Finally, the *neocortex* arrived on the scene,[13] a thin mantle hugging the brain and wrinkled in walnutlike convolutions. The cortical mantle has its own intricate organization. It consists of six layers, each characterized by its own neuronal composition. Certain parts of the neocortex are organized into vertical "columns" cutting through the layers and representing distinct functional units. The arrival of the neocortex has radically changed the way information is processed and endowed the brain with far greater computational powers and complexity. The division into two lateral twin systems continues within the cortex, giving rise to two cerebral hemispheres. The distinction between the "perception" and "action" systems is also retained at the neocortical level, the posterior (back) part of the cortex dedicated to perception and the anterior part (front) dedicated to action. But despite these divisions, the neocortex is much more heavily interconnected than its subcortical predecessors. As we will see later, this may have been its adaptive raison d'être.

The arrival of the neocortex radically changed the "balance of power" within the brain. The ancient subcortical structures, which used to discharge certain functions independently, now found themselves subordinated to the neocortex and assumed supporting functions in the shadow of the new level of neural organization. For a scientist trying to understand these functions this presents a source of confusion: what these subcortical structures had evolved to do before the advent of the cortex is probably not exactly what they do today, in the fully cortical brain. And so, paradoxically, our understanding of cortical functions is in many respects more precise than our understanding of the thalamic or basal ganglia functions, despite the fact that the cortex is, in some sense, more "advanced."

The neocortex consists of distinct regions, called *cytoarchitechtonic regions,* each characterized by its own type of neuronal composition and patterns of local connectivity. The neocortex performs diverse functions, yet no simple relationship exists between its different functions and cytoarchitectonic regions. The neocortex consists of four major lobes, each linked to its own type of information. The *occipital* lobe deals with visual information, the *temporal* lobe deals with sounds, the *parietal* lobe deals with tactile sensations, and the *frontal* lobe deals with movements.

At a very late stage of cortical evolution, two major developments took place: the emergence of language and a rapid ascent of the executive functions. As we will see, language acquires its place in the neocortex by attaching itself to various cortical areas in a highly distributed way. And the executive functions emerge as the brain's command post in the front portion of the frontal lobe, the *prefrontal cortex.* The frontal lobes undergo an explosive expansion at the late stage of evolution.

According to Korbinian Brodmann,[14] the prefrontal cortex or its analogues account for 29% of the total cortex in humans, 17% in the chimpanzee, 11.5% in the gibbon and the macaque, 8.5% in the lemur, 7% in the dog, and 3.5% in the cat (Fig. 4.1). There are several ways of delineating the prefrontal cortex relative to other cortical areas. One such method is based on so-called cytoarchitectonic maps, maps of the cortex comprised of morphologically distinct, numbered brain regions (Fig. 4.2). These cortical regions are called "Brodmann areas," named after the author of the most commonly used cytoarchitectonic map.[15] According to this definition, the prefrontal cortex consists of Brodmann areas 8, 9, 10, 11, 12, 13, 44, 45, 46, and 47.[16] The prefrontal cortex is characterized by the predominance of the so-called granular neural cells found mostly in layer IV.[17]

An alternative, but roughly equivalent method of outlining the prefrontal cortex is through its subcortical projections. A particular subcortical structure is commonly used for this purpose: the *dorsomedial thalamic nucleus,* which is, in a sense, the point of convergence,

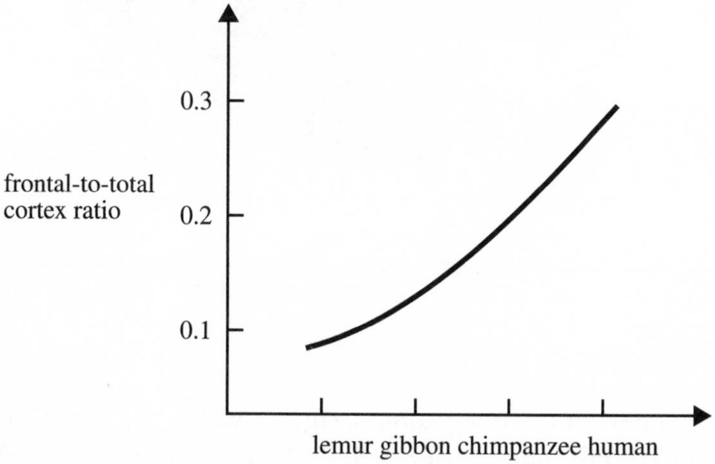

Figure 4.1. Frontal lobe ratio to the whole brain in different simian and primate species.

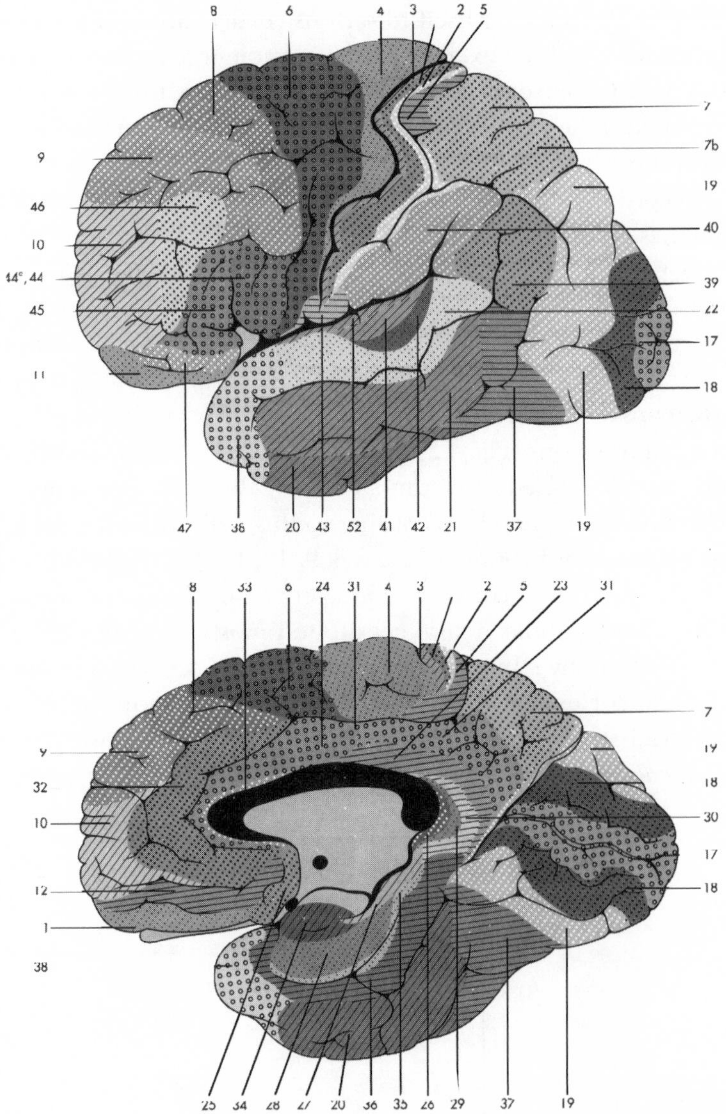

Figure 4.2. Cortical map with cytoarchitectonic regions after Brodmann. [Adapted from Roberts, Leigh, and Weinberger (1993). Reprinted with permission.]

the "summit" of the integration occurring within the specific thalamic nuclei. Prefrontal cortex is then defined as the area receiving projections from the dorsomedial thalamic nucleus. The prefrontal cortex is sometimes delineated also through its biochemical pathways. According to that definition, the prefrontal cortex is defined as the area receiving projections from the mesocortical dopamine system. The various methods of delineating the prefrontal cortex outline roughly identical territories. It is shown in Figure 4.3.

In a curious parallel between the evolution of the brain and the evolution of brain science (we will revisit the subject more than once), the interest in the prefrontal cortex was also late in coming. But then it gradually began to reveal its secrets to the great scientists and clinicians like Hughlings Jackson,[18] and Alexandr Luria,[19] and in the last few decades to researchers like Antonio Damasio,[20] Joaquin Fuster,[21] Patricia Goldman-Rakic,[22] and Donald Stuss and Frank Benson.[23]

The Command Post and Its Connections

A command post is only as good as its lines of communications with the combat units. True to its "executive" functions, the prefrontal cortex is probably the best-connected part of the brain. The prefrontal cortex is directly interconnected with every distinct functional unit of the brain.[24] It is connected to the posterior association cortex, the highest station of perceptual integration, and also with the premotor cortex, basal ganglia, and the cerebellum, all involved in various aspects of motor control and movements. The prefrontal cor-

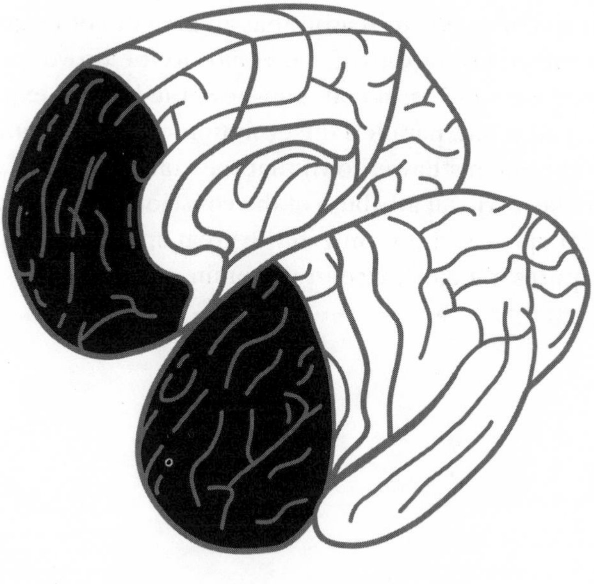

Figure 4.3. Prefrontal cortex.

tex is connected with the dorsomedial thalamic nucleus, the highest station of neural integration within the thalamus; with the hippocampus and related structures, known to be critical for memory; and with the cingulate cortex, presumed to be critical for emotion and dealing with uncertainty. In addition, this command post connects with the amygdala, which regulates most basic relations between the individual members of the species, and with the hypothalamus, in charge of control over the vital homeostatic functions. Last but far from least, it is connected with the brain stem nuclei in charge of activation and arousal.

Of all the structures in the brain, only the prefrontal cortex is embedded in such a richly networked pattern of neural pathways. This unique connectivity makes the frontal lobes singularly suited for coordinating and integrating the work of all the other brain structures—the conductor of the orchestra. As we shall later see, this extreme connectivity also puts the frontal lobes at particular risk for disease. As in political, economic, and military organizations, the leader is ultimately responsible for the subordinates' blunders.

We will see later that the prefrontal cortex, unique among the brain structures, seems to contain the map of the whole cortex, an assertion first made by Hughlings Jackson[25] at the end of the nineteenth century. This property of the prefrontal cortex may be the critical prerequisite of consciousness, the "inner perception." Since any aspect of our mental world may, in principle, be the focus of our consciousness, it stands to reason that an area of convergence of all its neural substrates must exist. This leads to the provocative proposition that the evolution of consciousness, the highest expression of the developed brain, parallels the evolution of the prefrontal cortex. Indeed, experiments have shown that the concept of "self," which is deemed to be a critical attribute of the conscious mind, appears only in the great apes. And it is only in the great apes that the prefrontal cortex acquires a major place in the brain.

5

The Orchestra's Front Row: The Cortex

Sounds and Players

To appreciate the role of the conductor, one must recognize the complexity of the orchestra. The brain orchestra consists of a large collection of players—the skills, competencies, and knowledge that comprise our mental world. And the neocortex indisputably includes the brain orchestra's most accomplished players.

Scientists have long been intrigued by the complexity and functional diversity of the brain, particularly its most advanced part, the cortex. Most of us have seen, in college textbooks or on junk-store shelves, old phrenological maps. Today they are mostly dismissed as bizarre quackery. Yet they reflect the state-of-the art understanding of brain organization around the early nineteenth century, when the father of phrenology, Franz Joseph Gall, published his influential work.[1] Phrenologists looked at the bumps on the surface of the skull and related them to individual mental abilities and personality traits. Of those relationships, they constructed elaborate maps placing specific mental attributes in specific parts of the brain.

From the standpoint of contemporary science, phrenological maps represented a false start. Like alchemy's relation to chemistry, phrenology belongs to the prehistory of neuroscience, rather than its early history. Yet it was the first time that the cortex was considered as an ensemble of distinct parts, an orchestra rather than a single instrument, and an attempt was made to identify the players. And the false start represented by phrenology highlighted a fundamental problem inherent in every field of inquiry, that of the relationship between the commonsense language of description and scientific language of analysis.

We are all in command of certain cognitive skills (reading, writing, computing), traits (courage, wisdom, recklessness), and attitudes (affection, contempt, hesitation). At first glance, the meaning of these words appears self-evident, and one might expect that each of these properties of the mind should have its distinct location in the brain. This was the dominant belief as recently as a century and a half ago, as the phrenological map in Figure 5.1 illustrates.

Scientists have since learned that the way everyday human language labels mental traits and behaviors does not quite correspond to the way they are represented in the brain. Today, we still think of the cortex as consisting of many functionally distinct parts. Yet the scientific language that we use to describe these distinct functions

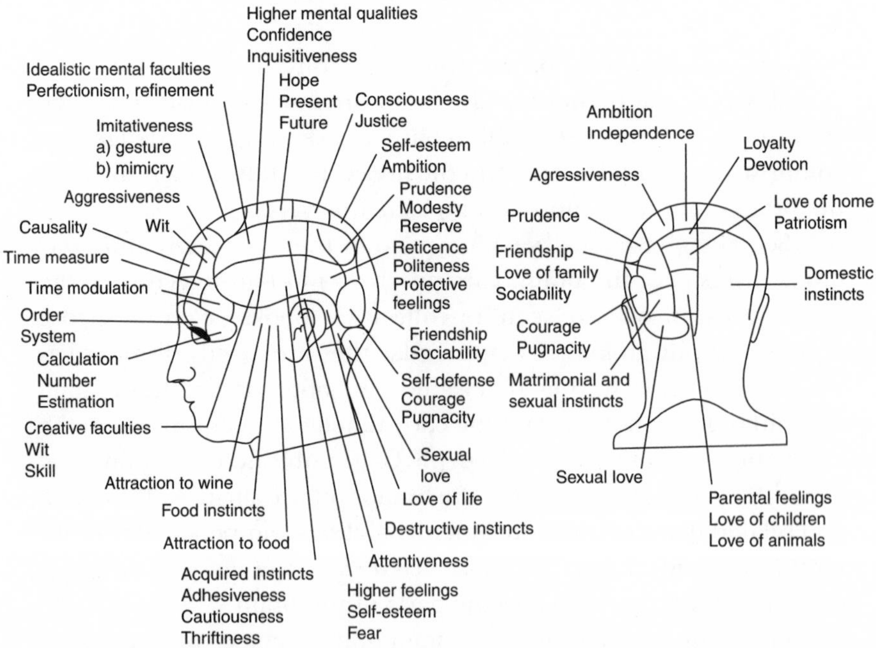

Figure 5.1. Phrenological map in the spirit of Gall. [From *Higher Cortical Functions in Man, Second Edition,* by A. R. Luria. Copyright © 1979 by Consultants Bureau Enterprises, Inc. and Basic Books, Inc. Reprinted by permission of Basic Books, a member of Perseus Books, L.L.C.]

has changed substantially. Just compare the two maps in Figures 5.1 and 5.2. The first brain map was designed by Gall at the beginning of the nineteenth century. The second brain map was designed by the famous neurologist Kleist at the beginning of the twentieth century.[2] While obviously not current, the second map is much closer to the principles of neural organization as we understand them today.

The change in our understanding of the brain is reflected in these two maps. The difference between them represents more than the incremental growth of knowledge. It represents a paradigmatic shift, which took approximately a century to complete. In every field of knowledge, a profound difference exists between the commonsense language and scientific language used to describe its domain. Everyday language describes the world in terms of tables, chairs, stones, rivers, flowers, and trees. Early belief systems, the ancient precursors of science, attempted to explain the world by postulating a separate deity for every such everyday object.

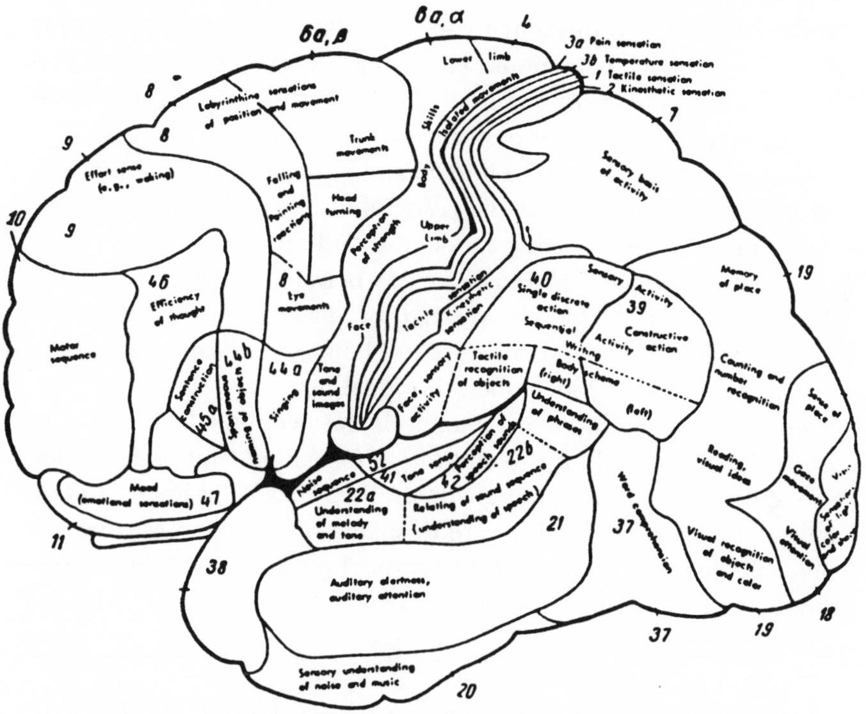

Figure 5.2. Cortical localization of functions after Kleist. [From *Higher Cortical Functions in Man, Second Edition,* by A. R. Luria. Copyright © 1979 by Consultants Bureau Enterprises, Inc. and Basic Books, Inc. Reprinted by permission of Basic Books, a member of Perseus Books, L.L.C.]

By contrast, scientific language describes the world in terms of units not necessarily apparent through simple observation. The language of physics describes the world in terms of atoms and subatomic particles; the scientific language of chemistry in molecular terms. Brain science is today where inorganic chemistry was in the days of Mendeleev, finding its organizing principles and working out the proper scientific language. The field is very much in flux. The transition from Gall's map to Kleist's map reflects this process. Phrenological traits like acquisitiveness, veneration, or self-esteem may make immediate common sense, but they do not correspond to distinct structures of the brain.

But what are the traits that do? Imagine yourself listening to complex music produced by an intricate array of unknown, and unseen, musical instruments, while trying to figure out what the instruments are, how many, and what each of them contributes to the totality of acoustic experience. You will hear loud tunes and quiet tunes, mellow tunes and piercing tunes, but how do these common-sense descriptions correspond to the actual composition of the orchestra? This is the challenge that generations of neuroscientists had to meet with limited and imprecise tools—a bit like the proverbial blind brahmins laboring to discern the nature of the elephant. The true "orchestra" of cognition is often difficult to understand in commonsense terms. Really, what do things like "tactile recognition" in Kleist's map have to do with our everyday feelings, thoughts, and actions?

Assuming that a relationship exists between structure and function, our quest is aided somewhat by distinct features of brain morphology. The cortex consists of two hemispheres, and each hemisphere consists of four lobes: occipital, parietal, temporal, and frontal. Traditionally, the occipital lobe has been linked to visual information, temporal lobe to auditory information, and parietal lobe to tactile information. The left hemisphere has been linked to language and the right hemisphere to spatial processing. Over the last decades, however, many of these entrenched beliefs have been challenged by new findings and theories.

Novelty, Routines, and Cerebral Hemispheres

That one hemisphere (in most cases, left) is more intimately linked to language than the other has been known for many years. Paul

Pierre Broca[3] and Carl Wernicke[4] demonstrated in the second half of the nineteenth century that isolated lesions of the left hemisphere drastically interfere with language. Aphasias (language disturbances) are commonly seen following left-hemispheric strokes but not right-hemispheric strokes.

The basic facts linking language to the left hemisphere are not in dispute. The question arises, however, whether the close association with language is the central attribute of the left hemisphere or a special case, a consequence of a more fundamental principle of brain organization. Any attempt to characterize the function of one hemisphere through language and the other through spatial processing leads to an unsettling conclusion. Since language, at least in its narrow definition, is a uniquely human attribute, any dichotomy based on language is applicable only to humans. Does this mean that no hemispheric specialization exists in animals? The scarcity of work on hemispheric specialization in nonhuman species suggests that this is still the prevailing assumption among neuroscientists.

But the assumption of human uniqueness of hemispheric specialization is counterintuitive, since we usually expect at least some degree of evolutionary continuity in traits. While many instances of evolutionary discontinuity undoubtedly exist, the working hypothesis in any scientific inquiry should be one of continuity. This was pointed out to me many years ago by none other than my own father, by profession an engineer, basically unschooled in psychology (and thus unencumbered with its preconceptions) but possessing general broad culture, rigorous logical mind, and common sense.

The assumption of human uniqueness of hemispheric specialization also flies in the face of our general belief in the relationship between structure and function. The two cerebral hemispheres are not mirror images of each other. The right frontal lobe is wider than, and protrudes over, the left frontal lobe. The left occipital lobe is wider than, and protrudes over, the right occipital lobe. This double asymmetry is called the *Yakovlevian torque*, after the prominent Harvard neuroanatomist P. Yakovlev, who discovered it.[5] The frontal cortex is thicker in the right hemisphere than the left hemisphere.[6] But the Yakovlevian torque is present already in fossil man, and many hemispheric asymmetries are present in the great apes.[7] Gender differences and hemispheric asymmetries in cortical thickness are present in the rat.[8] Planum temporale, a structure within the temporal lobe, is larger in the left hemisphere than in the right hemisphere in humans.[9] Traditionally, this asymmetry has been linked to language. Subsequent research has shown, however, that the sylvian fissure and in particular planum temporale, structures in the temporal lobe traditionally associated with language, are also asymmetric in orangutans, gorillas,[10] and chimpanzees,[11] just as they are in humans.

Brain biochemistry is also asymmetric. The neurotransmitter dopamine is somewhat more prevalent in the left hemisphere, and the neurotransmitter norepinephrine in the right hemisphere.[12] Neurohormonal estrogen receptors are more prevalent in the right hemisphere than left hemisphere.[13] These biochemical differences are already present in several nonhuman species.[14] In fetal monkeys androgen receptor concentration in the frontal lobes is asymmetric in males but symmetric in females.[15]

Thus it appears that the two hemispheres are different both structurally and biochemically in several animal species. It is therefore logical to suspect that the functions of the two hemispheres are also different in animals. But in animals these differences cannot be based on language, since animals do not possess language, at least not in its narrow definition! It is clear that a more fundamental distinction is needed to capture the difference between the functions of the two hemispheres. Ideally, it would not refute the association between language and the left hemisphere, but embrace it as a special case.

The idea that guided my approach to cerebral hemispheres was born 30 years ago in Moscow. As a student at the University of Moscow, I spent a lot of time at the Bourdenko Institute of Neurosurgery, where Luria had a laboratory. I became friendly with a few pediatric neurosurgeons, and over the bland fare of the hospital cafeteria they often spun their surgical tales. One tale sounded particularly puzzling. In very young children, I was told, damage to the right hemisphere was extremely devastating and damage to the left hemisphere was relatively inconsequential. Although these claims were not substantiated by formal research, they provided a hypothetical situation in need of explanation, an exercise in mental gymnastics I could not resist.

The claim was directly opposite to what is supposed to happen in an adult brain. In adults, the left hemisphere is frequently called the dominant hemisphere and is presumed to be particularly important. Neurosurgeons are often reluctant to operate on the left hemisphere for fear of affecting language. On the other hand, the right hemisphere is often presumed to be more expendable. In the old literature it was referred to as the "minor hemisphere." Neurosurgeons are generally more comfortable operating on the right hemisphere and electroconvulsive shock (ECT) is often administered to the right but not left hemisphere.

Is it possible that the left hemisphere is dedicated to language and is therefore "silent" until language is fully developed? That could possibly explain lack of adverse effect of left-hemispheric damage in children, but this could not explain the particularly severe adverse effect of right-hemispheric damage. Also, my neurosurgeon friends kept telling me that even when left-hemispheric damage affected the areas not commonly implicated in language, the consequences in children were quite benign.

It appeared that some sort of broad transfer of functions was taking place between the two hemispheres, from right to left, throughout development, and that this transfer was not limited to the acquisition of language. This gave rise to the idea that the difference between the two cerebral hemispheres revolves around the difference between cognitive novelty and cognitive routines. Is it possible that the right hemisphere is particularly adept at processing novel information and the left hemisphere is particularly adept at processing routinized, familiar information? I "imported" this idea with me when I moved to the United States in 1974. In 1981 my friend Louis Costa and I published a theoretical paper, for the first time linking the right hemisphere to cognitive novelty and the left hemisphere to cognitive routines.[16]

The Nobel Prize–winning psychologist Herbert Simon believes that learning involves the accumulation of easy-to-recognize patterns of all kinds.[17] Is it possible that the left hemisphere is the repository of such patterns?

Novelty and familiarity are the defining characteristics in the mental life of any creature capable of learning. In simple instinctive behaviors the triggering stimulus is instantly "familiar" and the degree of "familiarity" does not change with exposure. The organism's response is well formed from the outset and remains the same through the life span. The assumption is that the neural machinery controlling the stimulus response remains unaltered by experience. An example of such behavior is found in simple reflexes. When your nose itches, you scratch it automatically and unthinkingly. This response is not a result of learning and will not change throughout your life span.

The brains of higher animals, including humans, are endowed with a powerful capacity for learning. Unlike instinctive behavior, learning, by definition, is change. The organism encounters a situation for which it has no ready-made effective response. With repeated exposures to similar situations over time, appropriate response strategies emerge. The length of time, or the number of exposures required for the emergence of effective solutions, is vastly variable. The process is sometimes condensed in a single exposure (the so-called Aha! reaction). But invariably, the transition is from an absence of effective behavior to the emergence of effective behavior. This process is called "learning" and the emergent (or taught) behavior is called "learned behavior." At an early stage of every learning process the organism is faced with "novelty," and the end stage of the learning process can be thought of as "routinization" or "familiarity." The transition from novelty to routinization is the universal cycle of our inner world. It is the rhythm of our mental processes unfolding on various time scales.

The role of learning and learned behaviors increases throughout evolution, at the relative expense of instinctive behaviors. Is it possible that the emergence of structural and chemical differences between the two hemispheres was driven by the evolutionary pressures to enhance learning? Is it possible, in other words, that the existence of two different, separate but interconnected systems, one for novelty and the other one for routines, facilitates learning?

An experimental answer to this question would require comparing the learning abilities of two types of organisms: with and without two hemispheres, but otherwise of equal complexity. Since hemispheric duality is a universal attribute of all the advanced species, the experiment will never be staged. The best the investigator might be able to do is to plot the evolutionary growth curves of learning abilities and of hemispheric differentiation, hoping to see a parallel. But plotting such "curves" is an imprecise enterprise, based on arbitrary assumptions.

The arsenal of science, though, is not limited to experimental and empirical methods. While still the mainstay of science, experimental methods are intrinsically limited. This is why most developed disciplines acquire their theoretical arm. A theory is a simplified model of some aspect of reality, which is usually constructed in a formal, often mathematical, language. Instead of direct experimentation, a model can be examined formally, or computationally, by deducing some of its properties from other properties. With the advent of powerful computers, it has become possible to combine deductive and experimental methods in a single computational approach. A model of the object in question is created in the form of a computer program, which is then actually run on the computer, simulating behavior. In this way experiments can be designed with the model, and the dynamic properties of the model can be examined through studying its actual behavior. Of all the new developments in cognitive neuroscience, the advent of computational methods is particularly promising.

Especially exciting among them are formal neural nets. Composed of large ensembles of relatively simple units, neural nets are extremely brainlike. They can accumulate and store information about their environment ("inputs"), providing that they get feedback about their behavior. They truly learn.

Neural nets are being used increasingly to model and better understand the processes in the real brain. Stephen Grossberg, one of the pioneers of neural-net modeling, discovered that the computational efficiency is indeed enhanced by the splitting of the system into two parts, one dealing with novel inputs and the other with routine inputs.[18] Other computational theories have also recognized the distinction between the exploratory behavior in novel situations and cognitive routines in stationary situations. Although none of these theories explicitly linked these two processes to the two cerebral hemispheres, they provided an additional argument that the emergence of such a split in evolution would confer a computational advantage on the brain.

Linking novelty to the right hemisphere and cognitive routines to the left hemisphere forces an entirely new way of looking at the brain. The traditional understanding of hemispheric roles in cognition has been static and generic. Certain functions, like language, were thought to be invariably linked to the left hemisphere. Other functions, like spatial processing, were presumed to be linked to the right hemisphere in an equally inviolable fashion. A standard textbook on neuropsychology or behavioral neurology lists a fixed mapping of function into structure without much regard for any dynamic changes in the nature of this mapping. What happened to the old Heraclitian wisdom that "it is impossible to step into the same river twice"? Honored in most branches of neurobiology, this seemingly self-evident truth was ignored in neuropsychology for many years.

Furthermore, traditional neuropsychology and behavioral neurology tacitly assume that functional mapping of the brain is the same in all individuals, regardless of their education, vocation, or life experience. But this too defies common sense. Can a portrait photographer and a musician be using exactly the same parts of the brain to look at faces and listen to music?

Novelty and routinization are relative, however. What is novel for me today will become routine tomorrow, in a month, or in a year. Therefore, the relationship between the two hemispheres must be dynamic, characterized by a gradual shift of the locus of cognitive control over a task from the right hemisphere to the left hemisphere. Furthermore, what is novel to me may be familiar to you, and vice versa. Therefore, the functional relationship between the two hemispheres is somewhat different in different people.

By the right-to-left information transfer I do not mean a literal transposition of information. More likely, mental representations develop interactively in both hemispheres, but the rates of their formation differ. They form more rapidly in the right hemisphere at early stages of learning a cognitive skill, but the relative rate reverses in favor of the left hemisphere at the late stages. How these functional differences between the two hemispheres may emerge as a consequence of the neuroanatomical differences between the two hemispheres is discussed elsewhere.[19,20]

Depending on education, vocation, and life history, what is novel for one individual is routine for another. Therefore, the roles of the two hemispheres in cognition are dynamic, relative, and individualized. After all, the old Heraclitian wisdom does apply to the way the two cerebral hemispheres interact, just as it applies to every other branch of neurobiology. And even more important, the distinction between novelty and routinization can be applied to any creature capable of learning, and hemispheric differences based on this distinction may already exist in nonhuman species. At least this possibility can be experimentally explored and the evolutionary continuity across species ascertained. This is by far a more compelling framework of scientific inquiry.

The history of science is replete with false starts. Scientific progress, however, is not based on a wholesale refutation of old claims with the arrival of new ones. This indeed would have meant hopelessly circular movement. It is more constructive when a new theory or discovery embraces old knowledge as a special case under a more general concept. The novelty–routinization theory of hemispheric specialization does not imply that the traditional notions linking language to the left hemisphere are wrong. Instead, it embraces them as a special case of a uniquely human way of representing information through a well-articulated routinized code, language.

In science even the most plausible and aesthetically appealing hypothesis must be put to an empirical test. Much of the evidence to support the dynamic relationship between the two hemispheres was obtained with rather simple tools. These tools exploited the basic properties of neural wiring. The majority of sensory pathways in the brain are crossed: information from the left half of the outside world is delivered primarily to the right hemisphere, and information from the right half of the outside world is delivered primarily to the left hemisphere. This is true for tactile, visual, and to a lesser extent acoustic information. Of course, under normal circumstances the two hemispheres interact and share information owing to the massive fiber bundles connecting them, called the corpus callosum and the commissures. However, by delivering information very briefly to one side of the sensory field, it is possible to engage a single hemisphere, the one opposite to the side of the input.

This can be accomplished with rather simple devices. One of them, the tachistoscope, is a simple visual projection device exploiting this principle. For better or worse, the tachistoscope is probably responsible for more information about the workings of the two hemispheres than any other method. For acoustic information this was accomplished with a dichotic listening device, essentially a tape deck with two earphones.[21]

Much of the research with these methods revolved around the restatement and elaboration of the tired old static concept about the roles of the two hemispheres. Precious few breakthroughs were made. Most research was aimed merely at extending the laundry lists of left-hemispheric functions and right-hemispheric functions. However, some of the findings led to provocatively unexpected conclusions, which violated the established "truth." Music processing and perception of faces figure prominently on the right-hemispheric list. Prosopagnosia (impairment of facial recognition) and amusia (impairment of melody recognition) have been traditionally regarded as symptoms of right-hemispheric damage following stroke or other conditions. Yet the classic experiment by Bever and Chiarello demonstrated a striking relationship between the side of musical processing and musical expertise.[22] True enough, musically naive people process music mostly with the right hemisphere. Trained musicians, however, process music mostly with the left hemisphere. Since most people are musically naive, the old notion linking music to the right hemisphere is supported, but only in a weak, limited sense. The notion of an intrinsic, obligatory link between music and hemispheric specialization is no longer tenable. Instead, the side of processing musical information appears to be relative, determined by the degree of musical training and prior exposure to music. Similar findings have been reported for faces. Obscure faces are processed mostly by the right hemisphere, in keeping with the traditional views. But familiar faces are processed mostly by the left hemisphere.[23] Again we see relativity based on the novelty–routinization distinction!

Further confirmation of the novelty–routinization principle of hemispheric specialization comes from dynamic laboratory simulations of the learning process. Suppose a totally novel task is created, of the sort never experienced by the subject before and not even related to his prior experiences. Suppose, further, that the subject is getting extensive exposure to the task in a lengthy experiment extending over several hours or even days. Using the tachistoscopic and dichotic methods, it was possible to demonstrate that in the beginning the right hemisphere outperformed the left hemisphere. With repeated exposure to the task, however, the pattern was reversed, the left hemisphere emerging as the more accomplished one. The right-to-left shift of hemispheric control appears to be a universal phenomenon, which can be demonstrated for a broad range of learning tasks, nonverbal and verbal alike.

Compelling as the tachistoscopic and dichotic studies were, they required that the stimuli be presented under conditions bearing little resemblance to the way information is delivered in real life. The evidence was indirect, since it was inferred rather than directly observed in the brain. The evidence was also imprecise, since the tachistoscopic and dichotic methods are inherently incapable of revealing the exact neuroanatomy of information processing within the hemisphere. How relevant were these findings to real-life processes? It was important to demonstrate the dynamics of hemispheric interaction in more natural situations.

A dynamic theory of brain–behavior relations requires dynamic experimental tools. Truly appropriate research methodology to address the dynamic aspects of brain–behavior relations have become available only with the advent of functional neuroimaging. The dynamics of learning curves can be studied by imaging "snapshots" at various stages of the learning curve with much of the training taking place off-line between the snapshots.

A growing number of functional neuroimaging studies are using this methodology with modern technologies, such as functional magnetic resonance imaging (fMRI), positron emission tomography (PET), and single photon emission computerized tomography (SPECT). The evidence obtained with these methods also demonstrates an intimate link between the right hemisphere and novelty and between the left hemisphere and routinization.

Alex Martin and his colleagues at the National Institute of Mental Health provided a particularly compelling demonstration of this kind.[24] Using PET, they studied changes in blood flow patterns while subjects learned various types of information: meaningful words, nonsense words, real objects, and nonsense objects. Each type of information was presented twice, but each time with unique items. During the first presentation, when the task was novel, the right mesiotemporal structures were particularly activated, but this activation decreased during the second exposure. By contrast, the level of activation was constant in the left mesiotemporal structures. This is reflected in Figure 5.3. The findings are important, because blood flow level reflects the level of neural activation.

In Martin's study the right-to-left shift of activation was pervasive across all the four types of information, verbal and nonverbal

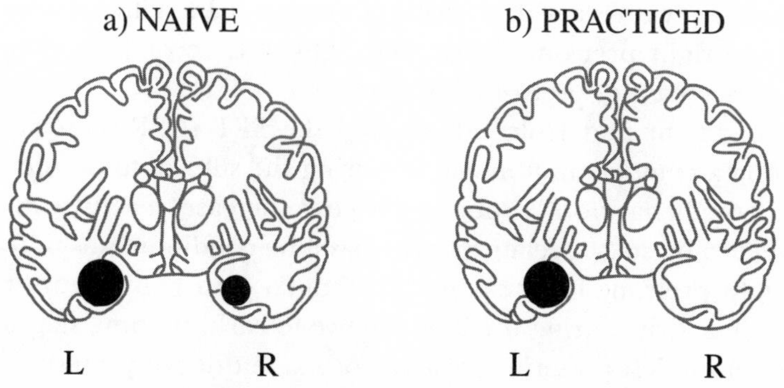

Figure 5.3. Changes in regional brain activation as a function of task familiarization. The right hemisphere is particularly active when the task is novel (a), but its activation decreases with practice (b). [Adapted from Martin, Wiggs, and Weisberg (1997). Reprinted by permission of Wiley-Liss, Inc. a subsidiary of John Wiley & Sons, Inc.]

alike. This means that the association of the right hemisphere with novelty and left hemisphere with routinization does not depend of the nature of information, but is universal. Furthermore, the right-to-left activation shift was present despite the fact that specific items were not repeated across the two successive trials. Thus the changes in the activation patterns reflect general aspects of learning, rather than specific item learning.

Similar findings have been reported by a group of British neuroscientists.[25] Both for faces and for symbols, exposure to unfamiliar stimuli was associated with an enhancement of right occipital (fusiform) activation. By contrast, increasing familiarity was associated with the decrease of right occipital activation and increase of left occipital activation. As in Martin's study, the novelty–familiarity effect is present regardless of the nature of the stimulus. It holds both for symbols (which in the orthodox scheme of things should be linked to the left hemisphere) and for faces (which in the orthodox scheme of things should be linked to the right hemisphere).

Using PET, Gold and his colleagues examined the changes in regional cerebral blood flow (rCBF) patterns in the course of learning a complex "frontal lobe" task (a combination of delayed response and delayed alternation) in healthy subjects.[26] Early (naive) and late (practiced) stages of the learning curve were compared. Frontal lobe activation was evident at both stages, but it was considerably greater at the early stage than at the late stage. Particularly noteworthy was the change of relative activation. At the early stage rCBF activation was greater in the right than left prefrontal regions. At the late stage the pattern was reversed, showing a greater rCBF activation of the left than right prefrontal structures. This was accompanied by an overall decrease of prefrontal activation.

Shadmehr and Holcomb studied the PET rCBF correlates of learning a complex motor skill requiring the subject to predict and master the behavior of a robotic device.[27] Increase of activity during early learning stages, relative to the baseline condition, was noted in the right prefrontal cortex (middle frontal gyrus). By contrast, increase in activity during the late, relative to early, training stages was noted in the left posterior parietal cortex, left dorsal premotor cortex, and right anterior cerebellar cortex.

Haier and his colleagues studied PET glucose metabolic rate (GMR) correlates of learning a popular spatial puzzle game (Tetris).[28] After four to eight weeks of daily practice on Tetris, GMR in cortical surface regions decreased despite a more than seven-fold improvement in performance. Subjects who improved their Tetris performance the most showed the largest GMR decreases after practice in several areas.

Berns, Cohen, and Mintun studied the PET rCBF correlates of learning, and relearning, rule-governed systems of relations ("grammars").[29] Grammar A was introduced first followed by Grammar B. The difference between the two grammars was too subtle for the subjects to be aware of the transition. Serial neuroimaging snapshots were taken in the course of learning Grammar A and then Grammar B. The learning of Grammar A was characterized by an initial surge of activation in the right ventral striatum, left premotor, and left anterior cingulate structures with subsequent decrease in activation. By contrast, a gradual increase of activation was noted in the right dorsolateral prefrontal and right posterior parietal regions. The introduction of Grammar B led to a second surge of activation in the left premotor, left anterior cingulate, and right ventral striatum regions, with subsequent decline.

Raichle and his colleagues studied PET rCBF correlates of a linguistic task (finding appropriate verbs for visually presented nouns).[30] A list of nouns was first introduced (naive condition) then, after considerable practice, replaced with a new list (novel condition). Naive performance was characterized by a particular activation of the anterior cingulate, left prefrontal, left temporal, and right cerebellar cortices. The activation virtually disappeared following practice and was partly restored during the novel condition, with the introduction of a new noun list. Additional analysis revealed prominent right cerebellar activation during the naive and novel conditions, but not after practice. By contrast, significant left medial occipital activation was present after practice, but not during the naive or novel conditions.

Tulving and his colleagues studied PET rCBF correlates of novelty and familiarity in facial recognition.[31] Familiarity was associated with the activation in a broad network of frontal and parieto-occipital regions bilaterally. Novelty was associated with the activation in a broad network of temporal, parietal, and occipital regions bilaterally. Additionally, novelty was associated with a distinctly asymmetric, right but not left, activation of the hippocampal and parahippocampal structures.

So we conclude that the body of evidence presents a cohesive picture, and that impressive consistency exists between the old "low-tech" tachistoscopic and dichotic methods and the state-of-the-art methods of functional neuroimaging. It appears that the cerebral orchestra is divided into two groups of players. Those sitting on the right of the aisle are quicker at basic mastery of the new repertoire, but in the long run, with due practice, those on the left of the aisle come closer to perfection. In the corporate analogy, the large organization that is the brain appears to consist of two major divisions: one dealing with relatively new projects, the other running established, ongoing production lines. In reality each cerebral hemisphere is involved in all the cognitive processes, but their *relative degree of involvement* varies according to the novelty–routinization principle.

The shift of the locus of cognitive control from the right to the left hemisphere occurs on many time scales: from minutes or hours, as in the experiments with within-experimental learning, to years and decades, as in learning complex skills and codes, including language. This shift may even be discerned on the scale transcending the life of an individual. It can be argued that the whole history of human civilization has been characterized by a relative shift of the cognitive emphasis from the right hemisphere to the left hemisphere owing to the accumulation of ready-made cognitive "templates" of various kinds. These cognitive templates are stored externally through various cultural means, including language, and are internalized by individuals in the course of learning as cognitive "prefabricates" of sorts. Any attempt to translate Vygotskian cultural–historical psychology[32] into neuroanatomical terms will inevitably lead to this conclusion. In a more poetic, metaphorical, vein, a somewhat similar conclusion was reached by Julian Jaynes in his rendition of the "bicameral mind" with the "voices of gods" emanating from the right hemisphere to guide our ancestors as they nagivated novel situations three millennia ago.[33]

Noah's Predicament and the Landscapes of the Brain

Over the last few decades, hemispheric specialization has become a trendy topic in popular literature. It is common to talk about "right-brain" and "left-brain" therapies, "right-brain" and "left-brain" traits, "right-brain" and "left-brain" personalities. But it is important to realize that the two hemispheres have much more in common than apart. The players sitting in similar positions on the two sides of the aisle play similar instruments. Hemispheric specialization is but two parallel variations on the same basic theme.

According to this theme, the occipital lobes are involved in vision, the temporal lobes in auditory perception, and the parietal lobes in tactile and somatosensory perception. But the human brain is more than a collection of narrowly dedicated sensory devices. We are able to recognize complex patterns, comprehend language, and analyze mathematical relationships. What is the neural basis of these and other complex mental functions? As we will see, the orchestra consists of many players whose contributions to the ensemble defy simple definitions and whose seating arrangement is both complex and fluid—truly a game of "musical chairs."

Neuroscientists have traditionally relied on the effects of brain lesions to understand how the normal brain works. In its most simplistic form, the logic of such inquiry goes as follows. Suppose damage to brain area A impairs cognitive function A′ but not cognitive functions B′, C′, or D′. By contrast, damage to area B impairs cognitive function B′ but not cognitive functions A′, C′, or D′; and so on. Then we may conclude that brain area A is responsible for cognitive function A′, brain area B for cognitive function B′, and so on.

The method is called the *principle of double dissociation.* This time-honored method is at the heart of classical neuropsychology. It has contributed to our understanding of complex relations between the brain and cognition more than any other method to date. However, it is flawed in more than one way. In a highly interactive brain, damage to one area may affect the workings of other areas. An injured brain undergoes various forms of natural reorganization ("plasticity"), which makes it a rather spurious model of normal function. Despite these flaws, the lesion method has provided a wealth of useful information about the brain and all our current theories of brain function are to some degree based on this information.

The effects of brain damage on cognition help answer not only the "where" questions, but also the "what" questions. By observing the multiple ways in which cognition may disintegrate, we begin to understand how nature "splits" mental functions into specific cognitive operations, and how these operations are mapped on the brain.

Over the last few years, the advent of powerful functional neuroimaging methods has changed the way cognitive neuroscience is done. As noted previously, these methods include positron emission tomography, single photon emission computerized tomography, and particularly functional magnetic resonance imaging. Based on various physical principles, from radioactive substance emission to local magnetic field changes, these methods have one thing in common. They allow us to observe directly the patterns of physiological activity in different parts of the brain as the subjects are engaged in various cognitive tasks. A prominent American psychologist, Michael Posner, likened the impact of functional neuroimaging on cognitive neuroscience to the impact of the telescope on astronomy. Just as the invention of the telescope at the beginning of the seventeenth century made direct observation of the macrocosm possible, the introduction of functional neuroimaging at the end of the twentieth century enabled us to directly observe the workings of the mind for the first time in history.

Functional neuroimaging has its limitations. Most of its methods do not measure neural activity directly. Instead, they involve proxy measures, or "markers": blood flow, glucose metabolism, and so on. Strong evidence exists, however, that these markers accurately reflect the levels of neural activity. Another limitation has to do with our ability to identify the sources of activation, relating different aspects of this activation to specific mental operations. Neuroscientists are developing increasingly powerful statistical methods for solving this problem.

Yet another problem is related to the relationship between task difficulty and task effortfulness, and the strength of the signal registered in the imaging device (fMRI, PET, or SPECT). With task familiarization and task mastery, signal strength usually drops.[34] In principle, this may mean that a highly automatic, effortless, "easy" task will fail to generate a detectable signal. But easy and effortless cognitive tasks are not, so to speak, extracranial. They too occur within our heads, and brain lesions continue to affect them. In fact, the *majority* of our mental processes are effortless and automatic, conducted, as it were, on autopilot. By contrast, the effortful and consciously controlled cognitive tasks represent only a minor portion of our mental life.

A real possibility exists that the currently available resolution of functional neuroimaging devices limits our imaging capability to the relatively "effortful" tasks, whereas "effortless" automatic tasks fail to generate a detectable signal. Most relatively complex cognitive activation tasks used in experiments probably consist of both effortful and effortless cognitive components. Therefore, their activation "landscapes" may be deceptive in that they reflect isolated peaks with invisible valleys in between. What you see may be far less than what you get. Trying to surmise the brain activation pattern of a cognitive task based on functional neuroimaging data may be like Noah trying to surmise the landscape of Mesopotamia after the Great Flood by staring at the peak of Mount Ararat protruding above the water. Understanding the relationship between signal strength and difficulty level in rigorously quantitative tasks will help interpret the fMRI and PET cognitive activation data. The available neuroimaging technologies are invaluable tools of cognitive neuroscience, as long as we are aware of their limitations and do not take the findings too uncritically and literally.

The introduction of new scientific methods is always exciting. At the same time, it threatens the stability of established assumptions. Most scientific discoveries expand and elaborate previously accumulated knowledge, rather than refuting it. The points of discontinuity in the flow of scientific progress are relatively rare. When they occur, and the old assumptions are refuted in favor of radically different ones, we say that a "paradigm shift" has taken place. The historians of science have hotly debated the relationship between the advances in scientific methods and conceptual breakthroughs. What drives what? Not every new scientific method, revolutionary though it may be, leads to an instant conceptual paradigm shift. The good news is that the recent functional neuroimaging findings have by and large confirmed the earlier insights based on lesion studies. The bad news is that major conceptual breakthroughs have yet to follow.

Module Madness

In the early 1980s Gall and his phrenology enjoyed an odd revival under the name of "modularity."[35] Brain lesions sometimes produce very particular and narrow cognitive deficits. They may affect the names of objects belonging to a specific category (e.g., flowers or animals) but spare all the other object names. Or they may impair the recognition of a specific class of objects but not other objects. For years, neuropsychologists have been enthralled by such phenomena, known as "strong dissociations." Some of the reported strong dissociations were uncanny. In one study a patient who was unable to name a peach or an orange had no difficulty naming an abacus and a sphinx!

Strong dissociations are rare and most clinicians encounter not a single such case in the course of their careers. Nonetheless, many scientists felt that strong dissociations were particularly interesting and informative for understanding the brain mechanisms of cognition. Neuropsychological discovery and theory building became extremely dependent on the search for such "interesting cases" and their theoretical value has become an article of faith. The large numbers of mundane cases necessary to sort through in order to extract the precious few strong dissociations were being dismissed as uninformative.

This circular pursuit has led to the conclusion that the cortex consists of distinct modules, each in charge of a highly specific cognitive function. The assumption was that the modules are encapsulated, separated by distinct borders and with very limited interactions. The cases with highly specific cognitive deficits were interpreted as the breakdown of narrowly dedicated modules, and the existence of such cases was taken as the proof of the existence of the modules.

In this scheme of things, the cortex is understood as a mosaic of numerous modules separated by distinct borders with restricted communications between them. Each module is invested with a highly specific function. Searching for strong dissociations was accepted as the foremost method of identifying the mysterious modules. For each newly reported strong dissociation a new module was postulated, and the list was growing. This was remarkably similar to the heyday of phrenology, except that the strong dissociations caused by brain lesions have replaced the bumps on the skull as the leading source of insight.

The fallacy of this approach becomes apparent if one realizes that for every case of strong dissociations there are hundreds of cases of weak dissociations, where many functions are impaired together, albeit to different degrees. By making an a priori decision that these far more numerous cases are unimportant and only the strong dissociations are important, one inevitably drifts toward a bias in favor of the modular model of the brain.

In reality, the modular theory explains very little, since by lacking the ability to reduce multitudes of specific facts to simplifying general principles it fails the basic requirement of any scientific theory. Like the belief systems of antiquity, it merely relabels its domain by inventing a new deity for each thing. Nonetheless, like every simplistic notion, it has the seductiveness and illusory appeal of instant explainability—by introducing a new module for every new observation!

Given the extreme rarity of strong dissociations, they are likely to reflect the idiosyncrasies of individual cognitive styles and backgrounds and to have little to do with the invariant principles of brain organization. If this is so, then the rare strong dissociations are nothing but uninterpretable statistical aberrations.

Consider the following: I am a native Russian speaker who learned English in my teens. My proficiency in both languages varies depending on the circumstances and is replete with strong dissociations. The effects of fatigue, inebriation, or illness have distinct, and opposite, effects on my ability to communicate in the two languages. In English my command of concrete lexicon (e.g., household objects, which I learned as a child) becomes very tentative, but my command of abstract lexicon (e.g., scientific terminology, which I learned as an adult) remains intact. In Russian the opposite happens: I begin to stumble in my attempts to convey high-level concepts but my everyday language remains invulnerable. Certain parts of the lexicon (e.g., names of flowers and fishes) are equally impaired in both languages, since I had never learned them in either. A good friend of mine, an eminent psychologist from southern California, is a native English speaker with an excellent command of Russian. He reports equally strong state-dependent dissociations, similar in character but not in specifics, in both languages.

Should either of us have the bad luck of suffering a stroke, cognitive neuropsychological theory may be affected differently, depending on which of us would be examined and in which language. Strong dissociations will be promptly documented and reported, all due to utterly idiosyncratic circumstances of our respective personal histories, absurdly irrelevant to anything of neuroscientific importance.

Arguably, bilingualism is relatively uncommon. However, other unusual cognitive factors may play a role in different individuals. In combination these exceptions may account for most strong dissociations. Every individual cognitive profile is a landscape consisting of peaks (strong points) and valleys (weak points), and the disparities in altitudes may be quite dramatic. My near-complete ignorance of fish and flower names in my native Russian language is a case in point.

The effect of an extensive neurological disorder on a vastly uneven cognitive landscape can be compared with a flood that submerges the valleys but spares the peaks. Graded differences between the individual strengths and weaknesses will assume the appearance of strong dissociations and the trusting neuropsychologist will be swept by the sea of artifacts.

Cognitive Gradients and Cognitive Hierarchies

A didactic ploy is often used to explain the organization of neocortex. The ploy is simplistic but heuristically powerful. It is based on the notion of a three-level hierarchy in the neocortex.

In the posterior aspect of the hemisphere, the first level of the hierarchy consists of primary sensory projection areas. They are organized in a "stimulotopic" fashion, which roughly means a point-to-point projection of the stimulus field into the cortical field. The projections are continuous (or as a mathematician would say, "homeomorphic"). This means that the adjacent points of the stimulus field project into the adjacent points of the cortical space. The primary sensory projection areas include the retinotopic visual cortex of the occipital lobe, the somatotopic somatosensory cortex of the parietal lobe, and the "frequencytopic" auditory cortex of the temporal lobe. In the frontal lobe, the first level of the hierarchy is represented by the motor cortex, which is also somatotopic. The mapping between the stimulus spaces and the primary projection areas is topologically correct but metrically distorted. Different cortical territories are allocated to different parts of the stimulus space not on the basis of their relative sizes, but on the basis of their relative importance.

The second level of the hierarchy consists of cortical areas which are involved in more complex information processing. These areas are no longer organized in a stimulotopic fashion. However, each of these areas is still linked to a particular modality. These cortical areas, called modality-specific association cortices, are adjacent to the primary projection cortical areas.

Finally, the third level of the hierarchy consists of the cortical regions that appear at the latest stages of the evolution of the brain and are presumed to be central to the most complex aspects of information processing. They are not linked to any single modality. Instead, the function of these cortical areas is to integrate the inputs coming from many modalities. They are called heteromodal association cortices and include the inferotemporal cortex, inferoparietal cortex, and of course the prefrontal cortex.

When the effects of brain lesions are examined realistically and without strident preconceptions, a very different from modular picture of the brain emerges. Damage to adjacent parts of the cortex produces similar, albeit not identical, cognitive deficits. This pattern implies that adjacent regions of the neocortex perform similar cognitive functions, and that a gradual transition from one cognitive function to another corresponds to a gradual, continuous trajectory along the cortical surface. The way cognition is distributed throughout the cortex is graduated and continuous, not modular and encapsulated. This pattern of organization, which I have labeled "gradiental," applies particularly to the heteromodal association cortex; probably less so to the modality-specific association cortex; and least of all to the primary projection cortex, which retains strongly modular properties.

The concept of the cognitive gradient first occurred to me in the late 1960s, when I began to take courses in neuropsychology. Together with other students, I was being exposed to a potpourri of neuropsychological syndromes, an endless and disparate laundry list. I began to feel that I needed an autodidactic device enabling me to organize these neuropsychological syndromes into a coherent, simplifying scheme. The gradiental model served this purpose admirably, since it allowed me to interpolate syndromes rather than memorize them by rote. Then I came to realize that the gradiental notion of cortical functional organization is also a powerful conceptual and explanatory tool in thinking about the brain and brain disorders, far more powerful than the prevailing at the time view of the cortex as consisting of discrete functional regions. Among other things, my gradients enabled me to accurately predict the effects of particular brain lesions before empirically observing these effects, and I enjoyed the game. It also helped explain how different parts of the neocortex acquired their functions. I began to think of my gradients as the neuropsychological analogue of the Mendeleev periodic table of elements.

The first person I shared my gradiental theory with was Ekhtibar Dzafarov from Baku (now the capital of independent Azerbaijan on the Caspian Sea). Ekhtibar, a fellow student a few years my junior at the Psychology Department of the Moscow State University, was a protégé of mine. A brilliant polymath and mathematical prodigy, Ekhtibar was a study in cultural contradictions. He had a creative and rigorous mind thoroughly at home with Western philosophy and literature, yet he retained his Eastern mores.

Through happenstance, I was probably responsible for Ekhtibar's admission to the university. Graduate students were often asked to interview freshmen applicants as part of the admissions procedure. The dean's office alerted us to the particular attraction the Psychology Department presumably held for "mentally unstable" applicants. In light of this concern and in the spirit of the culture in which we lived, we were instructed to watch out for "psychotic" applicants and to surreptitiously mark their files with a Magic Marker—a kiss of death for the applicant's dreams of Moscow University.

And so I was sitting one sweltering July afternoon in a non–air-conditioned office of the Moscow University old campus on Manezhnaya Square, forcing myself to listen to an inarticulate young lout across the desk, my attention wandering. Meanwhile, my friend Natasha Kalita at the adjacent desk was interviewing an impeccably dressed, lanky southerner with jet-black hair. The young man, appearing still in his teens, spoke excellent Russian but with an unmistakable accent of the Caucasus. As I began to eavesdrop on their conversation to relieve the boredom, the young southerner was talking about the Goedel theorem, while Natasha's increasingly glassy eyes betrayed total incomprehension. As the southerner moved on to the Turing machine, I saw Natasha's hand reach for the Magic Marker. But I already sensed a kindred spirit and very quickly told Natasha to swap. She took over my incoherent lout and I completed the interview with the young southerner.

I wrote a glowing review and Ekhtibar became a psychology freshman, probably the brightest in the department. Following that encounter he attached himself to me and saw me as his protector. We quickly developed intellectual respect for each other and became each other's audience for our more far-fetched ideas and theories.

When a few years later I was ready to leave the country, Ekhtibar flew from Moscow to Riga to say goodbye. We spent an evening in quiet conversation in the living room of my parents' third-floor apartment. As a persona non grata and a "traitor to my country," I suspected that the apartment was bugged, and so we made sure that the telephone (presumed by most Soviet citizens to be the most common device used for apartment bugging) was removed from the room and disabled. Many years later Ekhtibar told me that on his return from Riga he was summoned by the KGB (Komitet Gosudarstvennoi Bezopasnosti, Committee of State Security), questioned about his reasons for visiting me, and had the content of our farewell conversation recited to him in great detail as a proof of the KGB's omniscience. I have no idea how they taped us. I can only guess that a van was parked on the street next to the building, filled with eavesdropping equipment. Although I had few illusions left about my old country's rulers, I found the story mind-boggling, sad more than outrageous. I was not a prominent dissident; by any rational standard, I was a political nobody. Yet this is how resources were being spent in the country not known for its wealth barely a decade and a half before its final collapse under its own weight.

And so it was Ekhtibar to whom I first divulged my homespun gradiental theory, which deviated sharply from everything we were taught about the brain. This was done in style, over Georgian red wine at lunch, while beholding a sweeping panorama of Moscow from the rooftop restaurant of the Ministry of Defense Hotel next to the university campus, colloquially known among students as "the Pentagon." The choice of venue was ironic, since I was in the middle of evading, with Luria's connivance, the Soviet military draft, a rather dangerous endeavor in that time and place.

Ekhtibar was impressed and endorsed the idea. So I decided to take it higher up and the next day discussed it with Alexandr Romanovich. I had always thought of my gradiental model as a direct and immediate derivation from Luria's own approach to brain–behavior relations. But to my surprise he did not see it that way and basically dismissed it in favor of the more traditional "localizationist" premise. One of many good things about Luria was that it was possible to disagree with him in a scientific debate without risking the erosion of the personal relationship. Even when he did not share your ideas, he did not feel threatened by them. His attitude was never one of irritation; it ranged from enthusiasm to benign indifference, and this is precisely what it was this time.

I got to write up my gradiental theory only 15 years later, in 1986, when I was privileged to spend a year as a visiting scholar at the Institute for Advanced Studies of the Hebrew University of Jerusalem. When the journal article in which I introduced the concept of a cognitive "cortical gradient" was finally published in 1989[36] and then published again as a book chapter,[37] it was largely ignored.

The notion of modularity was too entrenched and simplistically appealing. But today modularity is in retreat and the gradiental view of the cerebral cortex is on the ascendancy. This, I believe, represents a true paradigm shift in cognitive neuroscience, and like every paradigm shift it entailed an uphill battle. In a remarkable essay, "Scotoma: Forgetting and Neglect in Science." Oliver Sacks likens the recent changes in our views about the brain to the paradigm shift in physics at the turn of the twentieth century.[38] That was the time when the Newtonian physics of discrete bodies was supplanted by the new physics of fields—electric, magnetic, and gravitational.

As I argue later in this book, the notion of modularity is not entirely misplaced. Modularity probably accurately captures an archaic principle of neural organization, which was supplanted later in evolution with the gradiental principle. If this is so, then an uncanny parallel exists between the evolution of the brain and the intellectual evolution of how we think about the brain. Both the evolution of the brain itself and the evolution of our theories about the brain were characterized by a paradigm shift from modular to interactive.

A Thing Is a Thing

The gradiental principle is best understood by examining two fundamental aspects of our mental world: perception and language. Consider two alternative ways in which the mental representations of things may be coded. In the first version, various categories of things (fruit, flowers, clothes, tools, etc.) are coded as separate "modules," each occupying a distinct, circumscribed location in the cortex. In the second version, the representation of every category of things is distributed according to its various sensory components: visual, tactile, auditory, and so on.

The first possibility will be consistent with the modular principle of cerebral organization. In fact, the proponents of this principle usually quote cases of perceptual or naming difficulties affecting specific, isolated categories of things. As noted earlier, such cases are extremely rare, but they exist. The second possibility will be consistent with the gradiental, continuous principle of cortical organization. To help decide which of the two alternatives is closer to truth, we turn to a peculiar class of neurological disorders called "associative agnosias."

Imagine walking into a department store. You find yourself surrounded by hundreds of objects, most of them unique in at least some respect. How likely is it that you have already seen that particular pattern on a tie, that particular cut of a dress, or that particular shape of a vase? You have probably not encountered the exact replicas of any of these objects before. Nonetheless, you will immediately recognize them as members of certain familiar categories: a tie, a dress, and a vase. Paradoxically, these objects are instantly familiar, despite the fact that, strictly speaking, they are novel.

Categorical perception, the ability to identify unique exemplars as members of generic categories, is a fundamental cognitive ability without which we would have been unable to navigate the world around us. We take this ability for granted, and in most cases we exercise it automatically, effortlessly, and instantaneously. But in brain disease this fundamental ability may become severely impaired, even when the basic senses (vision, audition, touch) are unaffected. We call such conditions associative agnosias.[39]

Our knowledge of the outside world is multimedia in nature. We can evoke the visual image of the tree's green crown as well as the sound of the leaves ruffled by the wind, the scent of its flowers in bloom, and the rough feel of the bark under our fingers. How does the ability to recognize common objects suffer in associative agnosias? Do the various attributes of the mental representation of an object share a similar fate? Does the perceptual breakdown in associative agnosias occur according to whole objects or according to its sensory dimensions?

Research into the effects of brain damage on cognition has shown that in agnosias the ability to perceive objects is never destroyed completely. It is usually limited to certain sensory systems without affecting the others. Consequently, different partial agnosias have been identified and named. A patient with "visual object agnosia" is unable to recognize a common object visually but will immediately recognize it on touch. A patient with "pure object astereognosia" is unable to recognize the same common object on touch but will recognize it visually. A patient with "associative auditory agnosia" is unable to recognize a common object by its characteristic sound (e.g., a dog by its barking) but will have no trouble recognizing it either visually or by touch.[40]

So none of these forms of agnosia eliminates our ability to perceive an object completely, but only partially. In each form of agnosia, the deficit is usually limited to a distinct sensory modality (visual, auditory, or tactile); and in that and only that modality is the patient's perception severely impaired. By the same token, this partial deficit is usually not limited to a particular class of objects (like items of clothing or household tools) but affects all types of objects to some degree. Yet the patient is not blind, deaf, or numb. While the agnosias are definitely linked to particular sensory systems, sensations are not themselves affected. The deficit is one of the interpretation of sensory information, rather than of its reception.

What is the neuroanatomy of associative agnosias? The cortical territories whose damage leads to these agnosias are adjacent to the areas in charge of sensory inputs as they arrive in the cortex. The territory of visual object agnosia abuts the visual cortex of the occipital lobe, the territory of associative auditory agnosia abuts the auditory cortex of the temporal lobe, and the territory of pure object astereognosia abuts the somatosensory cortex of the parietal lobe.

From this it follows that the mental representation of a thing is not modular. It is distributed, since its different sensory components are represented in different parts of the cortex. And it is gradiental, since the regions of these partial representations are continuous upon the areas of corresponding sensory modalities.

A Word to a Thing

Consider two alternative ways in which the knowledge of word meaning may be coded in the brain:

1. Representation of word meanings is modular in nature. All the word meanings are bundled together and separated from the cerebral representation of the real physical world that they denote.
2. Representation of word meanings is distributed. It is distributed in close neuroanatomical proximity to the cerebral representations of the corresponding aspects of the physical world. This would mean that the meanings of different types of words are coded in different parts of the cortex.

Although most representations of things and events involve multiple sensory modalities, some are more dependent on certain sensory modalities than on others. In humans, mental representations of physical objects depend mostly on the visual modality and only secondarily on other sensory modalities. This is reflected in the idiom "to bring an image before the mind's eye"—not the "mind's ear" or the "mind's nose." You can test this yourself by asking a friend to describe a common object. The odds are that the description will focus on what the object looks like and only later, when pressed, on what it sounds, smells, and feels like. By contrast, a talking dog (a relatively more olfactory creature) would have almost certainly invented the idiom "to bring before the mind's nose." At the same time, mental representations of physical actions—walking, running, hitting—are less visual and more motor and tactile/proprioceptive in nature.

Objects are represented in the language by nouns, and not just any nouns but concrete nouns. "Chair" is an object word, but "independence" is not. Actions are represented in the language by verbs, specifically by concrete verbs. "Run" is an action word, but "equivocate" is not. What are the cortical representations of object words and action words like? Are they represented together in a distinct part of the cortex, or are their representations distributed, according to their meaning, throughout different parts of the cortex?

Lesion studies of patients suggest that the cortical mapping of language is decidedly distributed. The breakdown of naming is usually not global but partial. The loss of object words (or "anomia for nouns") is caused by damage to the part of the temporal lobe adjacent to the visual occipital lobe. In these cases action words are relatively spared. By contrast, the loss of action words (or "anomia for verbs") is caused by damage to the frontal lobe, just in front of the motor cortex. This suggests that the cortical representation of object words is closely linked to the cortical representation of objects themselves and the cortical representation of action words is closely linked to the cortical representation of actions themselves.[41]

Recent studies with healthy subjects using functional neuroimaging methods support this conclusion. Alex Martin and his colleagues at the National Institute of Mental Health reviewed a large number of such studies and concluded that both the cortical representation of objects and the cortical representation of word meanings denoting objects are highly distributed.[42] Various features of these representations are stored close to the sensory and motor areas that participated in acquiring information about these objects.

For instance, naming animals activated the left occipital areas, whereas naming tools activated the left premotor regions in charge of right hand movements.[43] This is depicted in Figure 5.4.

Again, a decidedly nonmodular, distributed, and continuous picture of cortical functional organization arises, consistent with the gradiental model. The knowledge of word meaning is not stored in the brain as a separate, compact module. Different aspects of word meaning are distributed in close relationship to those aspects of physical reality which they denote.

a) ANIMALS

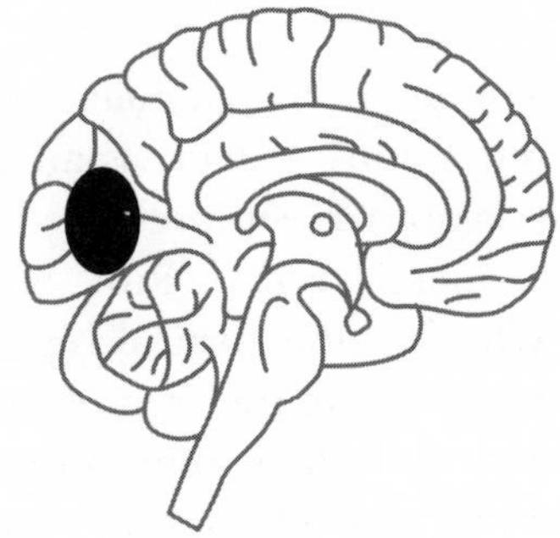

b) TOOLS

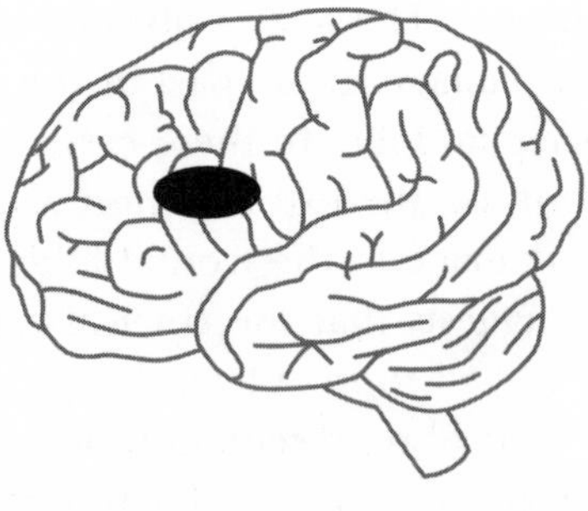

Figure 5.4. Distributed cortical representation of language. The cortical representation of word meanings denoting the objects are highly distributed. Various features of these representations are stored close to those sensory and motor areas that participated in acquiring information about the objects. (a) Area of increased blood flow when subjects name drawings of animals compared to naming tools. (b) Area of increased blood flow when subjects name drawings of tools compared to naming animals. [Adapted from Martin, Wiggs, Ungerleider, and Haxby (1996). Reprinted by permission from *Nature*, copyright © 1996 by Macmillan Magazines Ltd.]

Paradoxically, some of the findings commonly quoted by the proponents of modularity fit more naturally into the gradiental model of the cortex. The ability to name living things is more likely to be lost following brain damage than the ability to name inanimate objects.[44] Of all the findings mentioned in support of the modular view of the brain, this one is among the most robust and replicable. Yet simple common sense suggests a different explanation.

Most inanimate objects we come into contact with are man-made. Man-made objects are created for a purpose; we do things with them. In most cases, this implies that the mental representations of inanimate objects have an additional aspect: the representation of actions implicit in the objects. This aspect is for the most part absent in the mental representations of living things. As a result, the mental representations of inanimate things are more widely distributed, involve more parts of the brain, and are therefore less vulnerable to the effects of brain damage.

Like the mental representations of the physical world itself, the mental representation of language *denoting* the physical world is distributed. A close relationship, in fact a close parallelism, exists between these two neural records. They seem to be coupled, one attached to the other. This makes both evolutionary and (pardon the teleological impulse) aesthetic sense. The neural blueprint is both parsimonious and elegant.

6

The Conductor: A Closer Look at the Frontal Lobes

Novelty and the Frontal Lobes

The repertoire of every orchestra or troupe consists of pieces that have been its mainstay for years as well as relatively new additions. Likewise the products manufactured by a company consist of older lines of products and relatively new ones. Which pieces (or products) require closer ongoing attention by the conductor/director (or the CEO)? Common sense suggests that that the less streamlined or rehearsed the activities, the less likely they are to be successfully accomplished "on autopilot." Therefore, the less rehearsed, more novel activities require closer direction from the leader.

Functional neuroimaging experiments by Raichle and his colleagues highlight the relationship between the frontal lobes and novelty very dramatically.[1] The researchers used positron emission tomography (PET) to study the relationship between regional cerebral blood flow levels and task novelty. When the task (saying an appropriate verb to a visually presented noun) was first introduced, the blood flow level in the frontal lobes reached its highest level. As the subjects' familiarization with the task increased, frontal lobe involvement all but disappeared. When a new task was introduced, generally resembling the first task but not exactly like it, frontal blood flow increased somewhat but did not quite reach its initial level (Fig. 6.1). There appears to be a strong relationship between the task novelty and blood flow level in the frontal lobes: it is highest when the task is novel, lowest when the task is familiar, and intermediate when the task is partly novel. To the extent that blood flow levels are correlated with neural activity (which most scientists believe to be the case), these experiments provide strong and direct evidence about the role of the frontal lobes in dealing with cognitive novelty.

You may recall that novelty is associated with the right hemisphere. Does this mean that the frontal lobes are more intimately involved with the workings of the right hemisphere than of the left hemisphere? It just may. The right frontal lobe is larger in the right hemisphere than in the left hemisphere. And while it is specious to draw overly direct parallels between structure and function, most scientists believe that more neural tissue implies greater computational capacity.

The special role played by the frontal lobes and the right hemisphere in dealing with novelty and by the left hemisphere in imple-

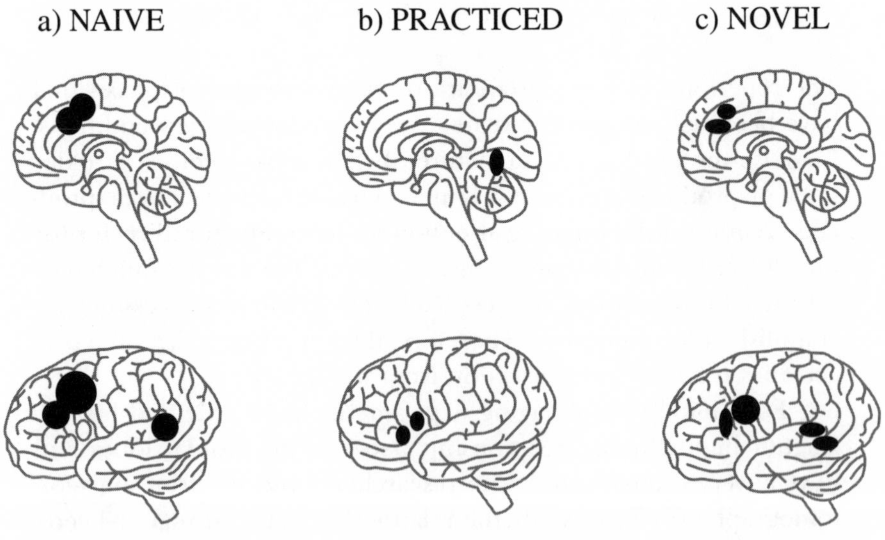

Figure 6.1. Frontal lobes and novelty. (a) The prefrontal cortex is active when the cognitive task is novel. (b) Frontal activation drops with task familiarization. (c) It becomes partially activated again when a somewhat different task is introduced, similar to the first one but not identical to it. [Adapted from Raichle et al. (1994). Reprinted with permission.]

menting routines suggests that the dynamic changes associated with learning are at least twofold. With learning, the locus of cognitive control shifts from the right hemisphere to the left hemisphere, and from the frontal to the posterior parts of the cortex.

This dual phenomenon, which I had described earlier, was dramatically demonstrated by Jim Gold and his colleagues at The National Institute of Mental Health.[2] Using PET, they studied changes in blood flow patterns in the course of performing a complex "delayed alternating response" task. Frontal lobe activation was very strong at the early (naive) stage and subsided considerably at the late (practiced) stage of learning the task. Its regional pattern had also changed. At the early learning stage the activation was greater in the right prefrontal regions than in the left. At the late stage the pattern was reversed: there was more activation in the left than right prefrontal regions. This is depicted in Figure 6.2.

In the old literature the right hemisphere was referred to as the "minor hemisphere" and the frontal lobes as the "silent lobes." Today we know that these structures are neither minor nor silent, although their functions may be elusive. The functions of the right hemisphere are less transparent than the functions of the left hemisphere, and the functions of the frontal lobes are less transparent than the functions of the posterior cortex precisely because they deal

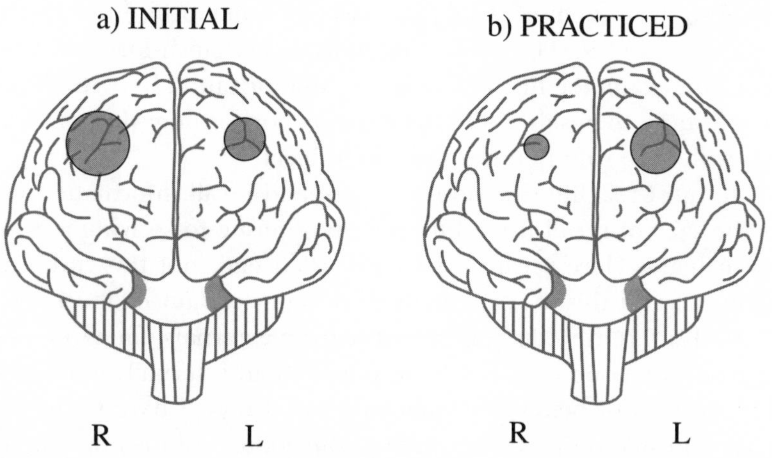

Figure 6.2. Frontal lobes, hemispheres and novelty. (a) A novel task activates predominantly the right prefrontal cortex. (b) As the task becomes familiar, the overall level of activation drops and shifts from the right to the left prefrontal regions. [Adapted from Gold et al. (1996). Reprinted with permission.]

with situations defying easy codification and reduction to an algorithm. So much for the minor hemisphere and the silent lobe! It took a longer time to appreciate their functions but now we are beginning to understand their true complexity and the central role they play in our mental processes.

Working Memory—or Working with Memory?

"Memory" does not sound like a mysterious concept to most people. In fact, the general public is so conditioned to the term that it is often used inclusively, and thus meaninglessly, to refer indiscriminately to every aspect of the mind. Ask ten people what "memory" does, and the answers will be pretty uniform: learning names, telephone numbers, the multiplication table, and cramming for the final test the dates of historical events you could do without. Memory is also among the most heavily studied aspects of the mind. In a typical memory study a subject is asked to memorize a list of words, a series of pictures of faces, and then to recall or recognize the material under various conditions.

Unfortunately, both the general public preconceptions about memory and the traditional ways of conducting memory research have very little to do with the way memory operates in real life. In a typical study of memory a subject is asked to memorize information and then recall it. The subject memorizes certain information because the examiner instructs him to. Memorization and recall are the end unto themselves and the decision concerning what to recall rests with the examiner, not with the subject.

In most real-life situations we store and recall information not for the sake of recall itself, but as a prerequisite for solving a problem at hand. Here recall is a means to an end, not the end. Furthermore, and this is particularly important, certain memories are accessed and retrieved not in response to an external command coming from someone else, but in response to an internally generated need. Instead of being told what to recall, I myself have to decide, which information is useful to me in the context of my ongoing activities at the moment.

All of us know all kinds of things. I know the location of barber shops on the West Side of Manhattan, the names of major Russian composers, the multiplication table, the main airports in Australia, the ages of my distant cousins, and on and on and on. How is it, then, that as I am sitting in front of my computer writing this book, I promptly access my knowledge about the frontal lobes and write about them, and not about the French Revolution or my favorite restaurants in New York? Furthermore, how is it that having gotten hungry after a few hours of strenuous typing, I equally promptly access my knowledge of neighborhood restaurants and no longer about the frontal lobes, that transition being seamless and instantaneous?

Most real-life acts of memory recall involve deciding what type of information is useful to me at the moment, and then selecting this information out of the huge totality of all the knowledge available. Furthermore, as the nature of our activities changes, we make a smooth, instantaneous switch from one selection to another, and then again and again. We make such decisions, selections, and transitions virtually every moment of our waking lives, most of the time automatically and effortlessly. But given the total amount of diverse information available to us at any given time, these decisions are anything but trivial. They require intricate neural computations, which are carried out by the frontal lobes. Memory based on such ever-changing, fluid decision, selection, and switches is guided by the frontal lobes and is called *working memory.* At every point of the process we need to access a particular type of information which represents but a tiny fraction of our total knowledge. Our ability to access it is like an instantaneous finding of a needle in a haystack, and it is nothing short of astounding.

Therein lies a crucial difference between a typical memory experiment and the way memory is used in real life. In real life, I have to make the decision what to remember. In a typical memory experiment the decision is made for me by the examiner: "Listen to these words and remember them." By shifting the decision-making process from the individual to the examiner, we remove the role of the frontal lobes and the memory task is no longer a working memory task. Most real-life acts of recall involve working memory and the frontal lobes, but most procedures used in memory research and to examine patients with memory disorders do not.

The disparity between the way memory is used and the way it is studied helps explain the confusion about the role of the frontal lobes in memory. An inconclusive debate on the subject has been going on for years, since the subject was first raised by Jacobsen[3] and Luria.[4] Recently, in large measure due to the work of the neuroscientists Patricia Goldman-Rakic[5] and Joaquin Fuster,[6] the role of the frontal lobes in memory has been reasserted and the concept of working memory gained prominence. Working memory is closely linked to the critical role the frontal lobes play in the temporal organization of behavior and in controlling the proper sequence in which various mental operations are enacted to meet the organism's objective.[7] Today the concept of working memory is among the trendiest in cognitive neuroscience. As is the case with trendy concepts, it is often used arbitrarily and loosely, which at times renders it meaningless. This is why it is particularly important to discuss this concept carefully and rigorously.

Since the selection of the information required to solve the problem at hand is made in the frontal lobes, they must "know," at least roughly, where in the brain this information is stored. This suggests that all the cortical regions are somehow represented in the frontal lobes, an assertion first made by Hughlings Jackson at the end of the nineteenth century.[8] Such representation is probably coarse, rather than specific, enabling the frontal lobes to know what type of information is stored where, but not the specific information itself. The frontal lobes then contact the appropriate parts of the brain and bring the memory (or as the scientists say, the "engram") "on-line," by activating the circuitry that embodies the engram. The analogy between the frontal lobes and the corporate chief executive officer comes handy again. Having signed a new contract, the CEO may have none of the technical skills required to do the project, but he knows who on his staff does and he has the ability to correctly select the employees for the project based on their particular expertise.

Since different stages of solving a problem may require different types of information, the frontal lobes must constantly, and rapidly, bring new engrams on-line, while letting go of the old ones. Furthermore, we must often make rapid transitions from one cognitive task to another, and to make things even more challenging we frequently deal with several problems in parallel. This highlights a very peculiar feature of working memory: its constantly and rapidly changing content. Imagine that you have five bank accounts with activities (deposits and withdrawals) taking place simultaneously and frequently. Imagine, further, that you have to keep track of the five balances in your head, without the benefit of a notebook or a computer, in order to run your business. Instead of memorizing a body of static information, you must be able to rapidly update the content of your memory all the time.

The five-account banking situation sounds pretty fantastic. But how different is it from the challenge facing a corporate executive, entrepreneur, mutual fund manager, political or military leader who must monitor, and act on, a number of situations rapidly unfolding in parallel? Now imagine a juggler with five balls in the air who has to keep track of all five constantly in motion. Now imagine mental juggling, which is what running a corporation, a business, or a scientific lab amounts to. This gives you an idea of what working memory does. With malfunctioning working memory, all the balls will soon be on the ground.

Let us now go back to our corporate executive. He needs to assemble a team of experts for a complex, long-term project with unforeseeable contingencies. At every stage of the projects he must identify the required expertise; decide how to locate the experts' names; actually find them; remember their names and telephone numbers at least for the duration of the project; identify the needs dictated by the next stage of the project; and so on. Imagine, further, that at every stage of the project he needs more than one type of expert, so that several parallel searches take place. This would be a reasonably accurate description of working memory. Working memory is very different from the activities we traditionally associate with the word "memory"—learning a fixed body of information and hanging on to it.

But the role of working memory is not restricted to large-scale decision making. We depend on working memory even in the most mundane situations. In your memory you have the telephone numbers of your favorite restaurant and of your dentist. You know where you keep your shoes and your vacuum cleaner. Even though this information is in your memory at all times, it is not the focus of your attention all the time. When you need to entertain your friends, you call your restaurant and not your dentist. When you are getting dressed in the morning, you go to the closet containing the shoes and not to the closet containing the vacuum cleaner. These seemingly trivial and effortless decisions also require working memory.

We have the ability to bring task-relevant information into focus as needed and then go on to the next bit of relevant information. The selection of task-appropriate information occurs automatically and effortlessly, and the smoothness of this selection is ensured by the frontal lobes. But patients at early stages of dementia often report "inane" actions. They may take dirty dishes to the bedroom instead of the kitchen, or open the refrigerator looking for gloves. This is an early breakdown of the frontal lobes' ability to select and bring on-line task-appropriate information. Working memory frequently suffers in early dementias. A person with severely impaired working memory will rapidly find himself in a state of hopeless confusion.

The paradox of working memory is that even though the frontal lobes are critical for accessing and activating task-relevant information, they do not themselves contain this information—other parts of the brain do. To demonstrate this relationship, Patricia Goldman-Rakic and her colleagues at Yale studied delayed responses in the monkey.[9] They recorded neurons in the monkey frontal lobes, which fire as long as an engram (memory trace) must be "held on" to but stop firing once the response has been initiated. These neurons are involved in keeping the engram on-line, but not in the storage of the engram.

Different parts of the prefrontal cortex are involved in different aspects of working memory, and a peculiar parallelism exists between the functional organization of the frontal lobes and the posterior cortical regions. It has been known for years that the primate (including human) visual system consists of two distinct components. The "what" system, extending along the occipitotemporal gradient, processes information about object identity. The "where" system, extending along the occipitoparietal gradient, processes information about object location. Presumably, visual spatial knowledge is also distributed. The memories for "what" are formed within the occipitotemporal system, and the memories for "where" within the occipitoparietal system.

Is *access* to these two types of visual memory controlled by the same frontal regions or by different ones? Susan Courtney and her colleagues at the National Institute of Mental Health answered the question in a PET experiment with an ingenious activation task.[10] A set of faces appeared in a four-by-six grid, followed by another set of faces. The subjects were asked to answer the "what" question (Are the faces the same?) or the "where" question (Did they appear in the same positions within the grid?). The two tasks produced two distinct patterns of activation within the frontal lobes, in the inferior portions for "what" and the superior portions for "where." Similar findings were obtained using single-cell recordings in monkeys by Patricia Goldman-Rakic and her colleagues at Yale.[11]

Apparently, different aspects of working memory are under the control of different regions within the frontal lobes. Does this mean that every part of the prefrontal cortex is linked to a particular system outside the frontal lobes? What happened to the conductor at large? Is there a part of the frontal lobes whose contribution is truly integral? Mysteriously, the area around the frontal poles, the furthest forward extension of the frontal lobe (Brodmann area 10), has so far eluded most attempts to characterize its function in specific terms. I would not be surprised if future research were to show that the areas immediately surrounding the frontal poles serve a particularly synthetic function and superimpose an additional level of neural hierarchy over the dorsolateral and orbitofrontal cortical regions. The synthetic functions probably played by this part of the brain are discussed in the next section.

Freedom of Choice, Ambiguity, and the Frontal Lobes

Consider the following everyday problems. (1) My checking account had the balance of $1000 and I withdrew $300. How much do I have left? (2) What shall I put on today: a blue jacket, a black jacket, or a gray jacket? (3) What is my dentist's telephone number? (4) Shall I go on vacation to the Caribbean, Hawaii, or Greece? (5) What is my boss's secretary's name? (I better get that one right!) (6) Shall I order lobster fra diavolo, lamb chops, or chicken Kiev for dinner? (My doctor says none of the above.)

Situations 1, 3, and 5 are deterministic. Each of them has a single correct solution intrinsic in the situation, all the other responses being false. By finding the correct solution—the "truth"—I engage in *veridical decision making*. Situations 2, 4, and 6 are inherently ambiguous. Neither has an intrinsically correct solution. I choose the lamb chops not because they are "intrinsically correct" (how ridiculous!), but because I like them. By making my choice, I engage in *adaptive decision making* (my doctor says maladaptive).

In school we are given a problem and must find the correct answer. Only one correct answer usually exists. The answer is hidden. The question is clear-cut. But most real-life situations, outside of the realm of narrow technical problems, are inherently ambiguous. The answer is hidden, and so is the question. Our purposes in life are general and vague. The "pursuit of happiness" is an amorphous notion meaning different things to different people, or even to the same person under different circumstances. At any given time, each of us must decide what the pursuit of happiness means here and now for me. In her famous retort to the question: "What is the answer?" Gertrude Stein captured this very well: "What is the question?"

We live in an ambiguous world. Aside from high school exams, college tests, and factual and computational trivia, most decisions we make in our everyday lives do not have intrinsically correct solutions. The choices we make are not inherent in the situations at hand. They are a complex interplay between the properties of the situations and our own properties, our aspirations, our doubts, and our histories. It is only logical to expect that the prefrontal cortex is central to such decision making, since it is the only part of the brain where the inputs from within the organism converge with the inputs from the outside world.

Finding solutions for deterministic situations is often accomplished algorithmically. It is increasingly delegated to various devices: calculators, computers, directories of all kinds. But making choices in the absence of inherently correct solutions remains, at least for now, a uniquely human territory. In a sense, the freedom of choice is possible only when ambiguity is present.

The absence of absolute algorithmically computable truths is precisely what sets leadership decisions apart from technical decisions. A conductor's or stage director's foremost responsibility is to provide an interpretation of a famous piece—an intrinsically subjective proposition. A corporate CEO makes strategic decisions in an ambiguous, fluid environment. Military genius is still regarded as the purview of art more than science.

Resolving ambiguity, or "disambiguating the situation" in scientific parlance, often means choosing the question first, that is, reducing the situation to a question which does have a single correct answer. In choosing the clothes to wear, there are many questions I may decide to ask: (1) Which jacket best matches the weather? (and choose the warmest jacket); (2) Which one is more fashionable? (and choose the newest jacket); (3) Which one is my favorite? (and choose the gray jacket). Precisely how I disambiguate the situation depends on my priorities at the moment, which themselves may change depending on the context. An inability to reduce ambiguity leads to vacillating, uncertain, inconsistent behavior. One is reminded of Buridan's jackass, standing in front of two haystacks and starving, unable to choose. Even the ancient Romans understood the perils of persistent ambiguity and coined the saying "Dura lex sed lex" ("Hard law is better than no law").

At the same time, an individual must have the flexibility to adopt different perspectives on the same situation at different times. The organism must be able to disambiguate the same situation in multiple ways and have the capacity to switch between them at will. Dealing with inherent ambiguity is among the foremost functions of the frontal lobes. In a sense, whether you are decisive or wishy-washy depends on how well your frontal lobes work. Studies have shown that patients with frontal lobe damage approach inherently ambiguous situations differently from the way healthy people do. The loss of the ability to make decisions is among the most common signs of early dementia. Damage to other parts of the brain does not seem to affect these processes.

In a nutshell, veridical decisions deal with "finding the truth," and adaptive, actor-centered decisions deal with choosing "what is good for me." Most "executive leadership" decisions are priority-based, are made in ambiguous environments, and are adaptive, rather than veridical, in nature. The cognitive processes involved in resolving ambiguous situations through priorities are very different from those involved in solving strictly deterministic situations. Ironically, cognitive ambiguity and priority-based decision making have been all but completely ignored in cognitive neuropsychology. This is not to say that other branches of psychology have ignored them. Projective tests like the Rorschach Inkblots have always been accorded a respected role in the psychodynamic tradition. But in its quest for precision and measurement, cognitive science has rejected such procedures as too vague, too subjective. Yet the lack of satisfactory scientific methods does not change the fact that priority-based, adaptive decision making in ambiguous situations is central to our lives, and that the frontal lobes are particularly important in such decision making. So rather than brushing the problem aside as "unworthy," the appropriate scientific methods must be found.

With my former graduate student Ken Podell, I tried to remedy the shortcoming with a simple experiment, using an original procedure called the Cognitive Bias Task (CBT).[12] A subject saw a geometric design (target), then two other designs appeared (choices), and the subject was asked to "look at the target and select the choice you like the most." (The CBT card is shown in Fig. 6.3.) We made clear to the subject that there are no intrinsically correct or incorrect responses, and that the choice is up to him or her. The experiment consisted of a large number of such trials, no two of them completely identical.

So the subjects were encouraged to do what they pleased. In reality, however, the designs were arranged in such a way that the subjects had two options: to base their response either on the properties of the targets (which changed from trial to trial) or on some stable preference unrelated to the target (e.g., favorite color or shape). Despite the seemingly loose nature of our experiment, the subjects' responses could be clearly quantified and were highly replicable. Our "cognitive projective" paradigm proved to be very informative, and we will return to it in several parts of this book.

We conducted our experiment with healthy individuals and with patients with various types of brain damage. Damage to the frontal lobes dramatically changed the nature of responses. Damage to other parts of the brain had very little or no effect. We repeated the experiment, but this time we disambiguated the task in two different ways. Instead of instructing the subjects to "Make the choice you like the best," we asked them to "Make the choice most similar to the target," and then to do it again, this time making the choice "most different from the target." In disambiguated conditions the effects of frontal lesions disappeared and the subjects with brain lesions could perform the task as well as the healthy controls (see Fig. 6.4).

Our experiment shows that the frontal lobes are critical in a free-choice situation, when *it is up to the subject to decide how to interpret an ambiguous situation.* Once the situation has been disambiguated for the subject and the task has been reduced to the computation of the only correct response possible, the input of the frontal lobes is no longer critical, even though all the other aspects of the task remain the same.

Of all the aspects of the human mind none are more intriguing than intentionality, volition, and free will. But these attributes of the human mind are fully at play only in situations affording multiple choices. We humans tend to claim the mental abilities we perceive as the most advanced to be uniquely ours. Numerous assertions have been made by philosophers and scientists that volition and intentionality are uniquely human traits. In its absolute form, this claim

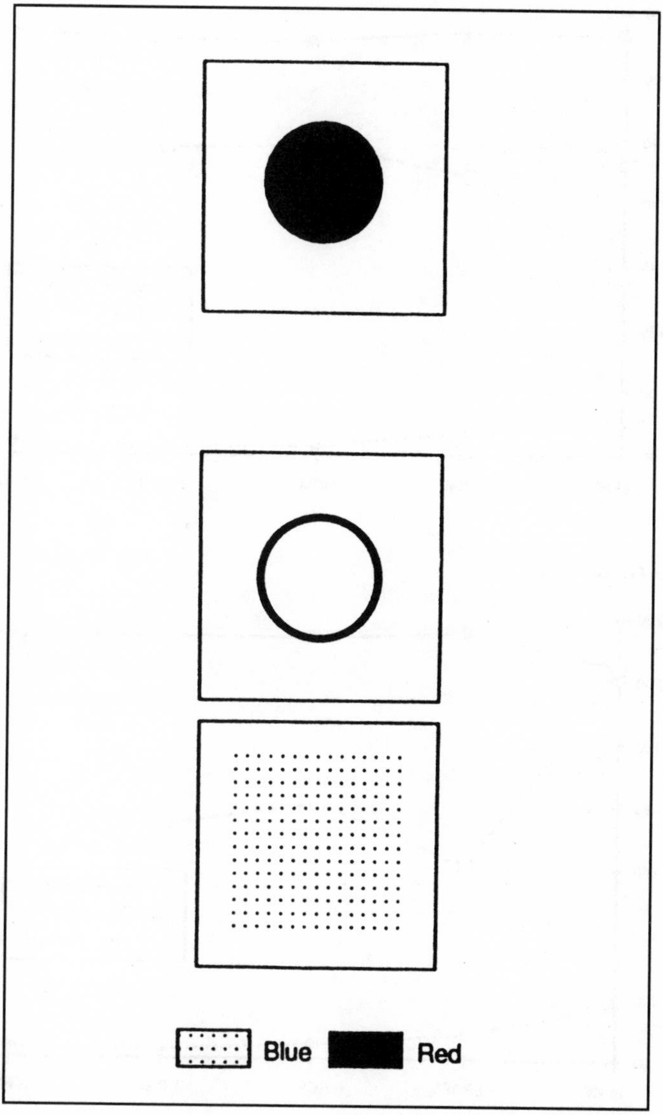

Figure 6.3. The Cognitive Bias Task (CBT). In the actor-centered version of CBT a subject is asked to look at the top form and then choose one of the two bottom forms that he or she likes most. In the veridical versions of CBT the subject is asked to look at the top form and then choose the bottom form more similar to it (or more different from it). Unbeknownst to the subject, one of the two bottom choices is always more similar to the target than the other one. [After Goldberg et al. (1994). © 1994 by the Massachusetts Institute of Technology. Reprinted with permission.]

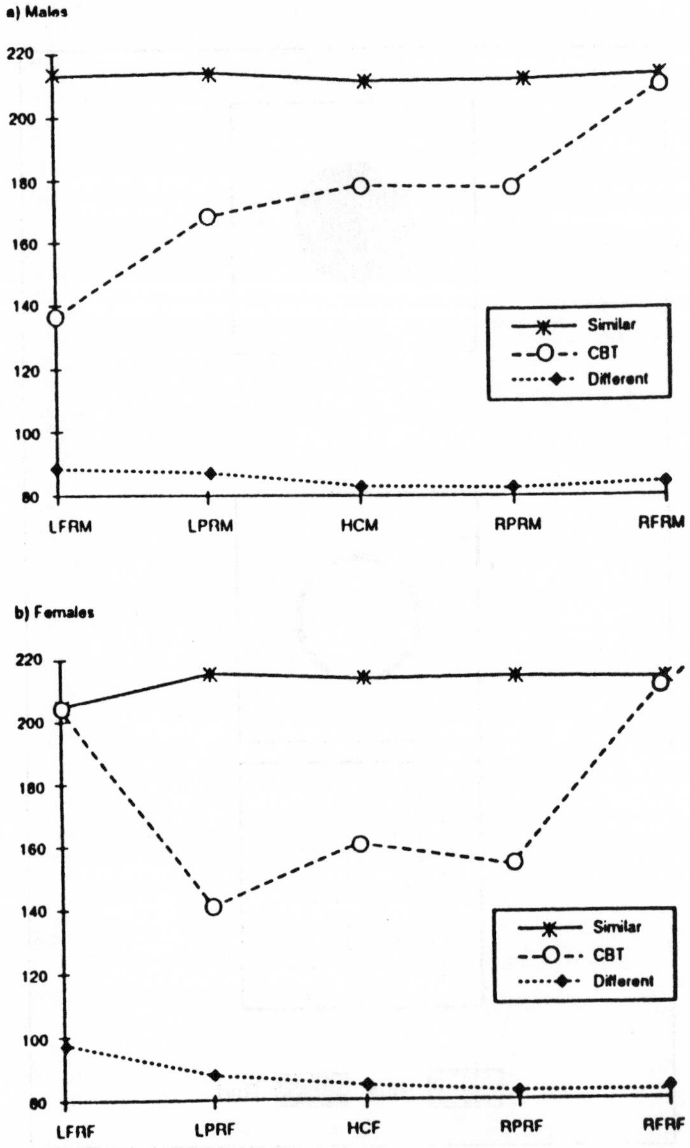

Figure 6.4. Actor-centered versus veridical versions of the Cognitive BiasTask. In the actor-centered version frontal lesions produce dramatic changes of performance on the CBT. The effects of lesions disappear in the two veridical versions of the CBT. This is true both for right-handed males (A) and for right-handed females (B). *Key*: LFRM, left frontal male lesion group; LPRM, left posterior male lesion group; HCM, healthy control male group; RPRM, right posterior male lesion group; RFRM, right frontal male lesion group. LFRF, left frontal female lesion group; LPRF, left posterior female lesion group; HCF, healthy control female group; RPRF, right posterior female lesion group; RFRF, right frontal female lesion group. [After Goldberg et al. (1994). © 1994 by the Massachusetts Institute of Technology. Reprinted with permission.]

cannot appeal to a rigorous neurobiologist. It is more likely that these properties of the mind have developed gradually through evolution, possibly following an exponential course. It is difficult to design a rigorous experiment to prove this, but an argument can be made that this process paralleled the development of the frontal lobes.

Cognitive neuroscientists are not the only ones who ignored actor-centered, adaptive decision making at their peril. Far worse, actor-centered decision making has also been ignored by educators. Our whole educational system is based on teaching veridical decision making. And this is true not just in the United States, but everywhere, at least within the Western cultural tradition. Strategies of actor-centered, adaptive decision making are simply not taught. Instead, they are acquired by each individual idiosyncratically, as a personal cognitive discovery, through trials and errors. Designing ways of explicitly teaching the principles of actor-centered problem solving is among the most worthy challenges for educators and school psychologists. Developmental psychology, too, focuses on veridical decision making, and the chronology and staging of actor-centered adaptive decision making is virtually unknown.

We do know, however, that adaptive decision making declines before veridical decision making at early stages of dementia. My former postdoctoral student Allan Kluger and I conducted a study at the Millhauser Dementia Research Center of New York University School of Medicine.[13] We compared the decline of performance on the Cognitive Bias Task and on its disambiguated, veridical analogue in patients at different stages of Alzheimer's-type dementia. Performance on the actor-centered, preference-based version of the task declined much earlier in the disease process than the performance on the veridical, "match-to-similarity" version. This is reflected in Figure 6.5 A and B.

This finding is important in more ways than one. It challenges the prevailing notion that the frontal lobes are relatively invulnerable in Alzheimer's type dementia. Most research suggests that Alzheimer's disease particularly affects the hippocampus and the neocortex.[14] It has been traditionally assumed that at the neocortical level the parietal lobes are particularly vulnerable in Alzheimer's disease and the frontal lobes less so. This well-entrenched assumption is probably a misconception caused by the systematic failure to recognize early cognitive symptoms of frontal lobe dysfunction as early signs of dementia. In fact, if you listen carefully to dementia patients and their family members, then it becomes obvious that

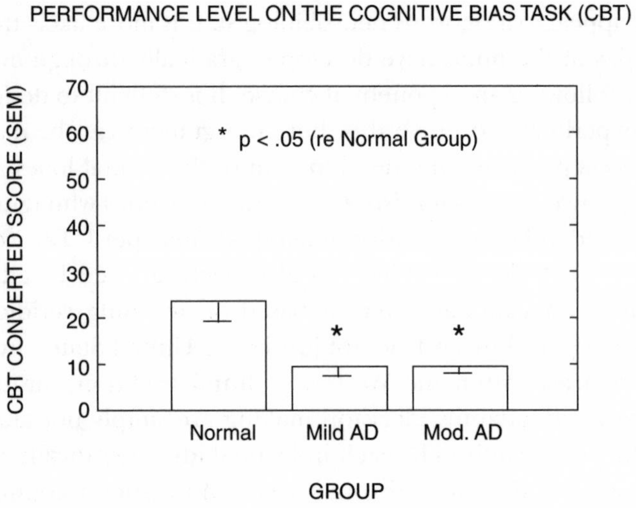

A

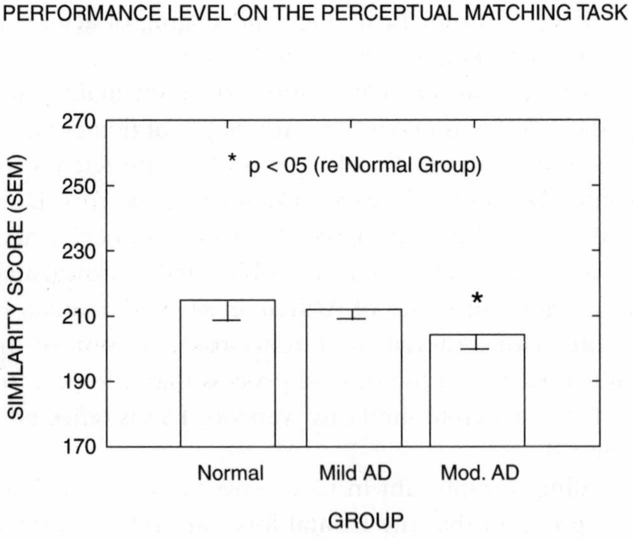

B

Figure 6.5. Actor-centered versus veridical decision making decline in dementia of Alzheimer's type. Actor-centered decision making declines at an earlier stage of disease process (A). Veridical decision-making begins to decline at a later stage (B). [After Goldberg et al. (1997).]

indecision, hesitation, and an increasing reliance on others for making choices are easily as common as memory impairment or word-finding difficulties at early stages of cognitive decline in the elderly. Unfortunately, the breakdown in actor-centered decision making is often misdiagnosed as depression or something else, often remaining completely unrecognized as a clinically significant symptom, an early symptom of frontal lobe dysfunction.

The search for highly sensitive cognitive signs of early dementia is a major challenge for clinicians, dementia researchers, and pharmaceutical companies. With the advent of new drugs for the treatment of dementia, a welcome and increasingly realistic prospect, it will become particularly important to have sensitive cognitive tools to measure the therapeutic effects of the new "cognotropic" drugs. The exceptional vulnerability of actor-centered decision making in brain disease offers an innovative strategy for developing cognitive markers of very early stages of dementia and highly sensitive tools for the assessment of cognotropic drug effects.

7

Different Lobes for Different Folks: Decision-Making Styles and the Frontal Lobes

The Neuropsychology of Individual Differences

Comparing the function of the normal and abnormal brain has been the mainstay of neuropsychology. It is, of course, understood that brain disease may take many forms, each corresponding to its own neurological or psychiatric condition: dementia, head injury, stroke, and so on. On the other hand, traditional neuropsychology and cognitive neuroscience have adopted an abstraction, the "normal brain," envisioned as a grand average of all individual brains. This simplistic notion has been frequently taken to an absurd extreme in many areas of cognitive neuroscience. This includes functional neuroimaging, the increasingly dominant methodology allowing scientists and clinicians to examine brain physiology and not just brain structure. The imaging data are fitted onto "Talairach space" (named after its inventor),[1] which is basically the brain of a single French woman, presumably selected on the assumption that its serves as a good approximation of all the other brains. To make things worse, only one hemisphere was selected and mirrored, ignoring all we know about hemispheric differences.

Neuroscientists are not unique in recognizing and appreciating the diversity of human minds, talents, and personalities as variations of normality. The world would indeed be a boring place were everyone the same and therefore to a large extent predictable. By noting that Joe Doe is mathematically gifted, musically inept, and short-tempered while Jane Blane is musically gifted, mathematically inept, and sweet, we do not automatically conclude that one is normal and the other abnormal. In most instances we assume that both are normal but different. A whole field of psychology has emerged to study the *individual differences as multiple expressions of normality.*

But does the brain have anything to do with these differences, or are they entirely a reflection of our different surroundings, upbringings, and experiences? Neuroanatomists have known for a long time that individual "normal" brains differ profoundly in overall size, relative sizes of different parts, and proportions. More recent findings suggest that individual brain biochemistry is also highly variable. These differences are particularly pronounced in the frontal lobes.[2]

Is there a relationship between the variability of human brains and the variability of human minds? In particular, are the differences in decision-making styles related to the differences in the anatomy and chemistry of the frontal lobes? We are only beginning to ask these questions, and by so doing, we are laying the grounds for a new discipline, the *neuropsychology of individual and group differences.* In due time, we may be able to understand the contribution of individual *neural* differences to individual *cognitive* differences. But the inquiry will proceed in steps, first by establishing this relationship with respect to groups rather than individuals.

Male and Female Cognitive Styles

Intuitively we understand that no individual cognitive landscape is a flat line. Instead, it consists of peaks and valleys, the peaks corresponding to individual strengths and the valleys to individual weaknesses. The quest for understanding the relationship between individual cognitive landscapes and individual brains drove the earliest attempts at mapping cortical functions, giving rise to the now discarded Gall's phrenology. In this tradition, individual cognitive differences have been understood in terms of who is better at what ("better" presumably corresponding to "bigger" in terms of regional cortical space).

Individual differences can be also approached in terms of cognitive *styles*, rather than cognitive *abilities*. Particularly, we can ask the questions about the individual differences in *decision-making styles*. This brings us back to the distinction between adaptive and veridical decision making made earlier in the book. If cognitive abilities influence the ease with which we acquire cognitive skills, then decision making styles influence the ways in which we deal with life situations as individuals. Most real-life situations of any degree of complexity do not contain a tacit unequivocal, single solution (the way the statement "2 + 2 = . . ." does). Placed into the same situation, different people will act in different ways; one is not unequivocally right and all the rest unequivocally wrong. How do we make our choices and what accounts for the differences in the ways we make them? Finally, what are the brain mechanisms responsible for the differences in decision-making styles?

My colleagues and I approached the question by giving our deliberately loosely designed Cognitive Bias Task (CBT) to neurologically healthy subjects.[3] You will recall that the subjects were shown three geometric forms (one target and two choices) and asked to look at the target and make the choice that they "liked the most" (see Fig. 6.3, a CBT card). It was clear that different subjects exhibited different response patterns. These response patterns gravitated toward one of two distinct strategies. Some subjects matched their choice to the target, and as the targets changed, so did their choices. We called this decision-making strategy *context-dependent*. Other subjects made their choices based on stable preferences, regardless of the target. They always picked blue, or red, or circle, or square. We called this decision-making strategy *context-independent*. To our surprise, males and females made their choices in strikingly different ways: males were more context-dependent and females were more context-independent (see Fig. 7.1). Although there was an overlap between the two curves, the sex differences were both robust and significant.

Gender differences in cognition is a relatively new and increasingly "hot" topic. For decades, neuroscientists treated humanity as a

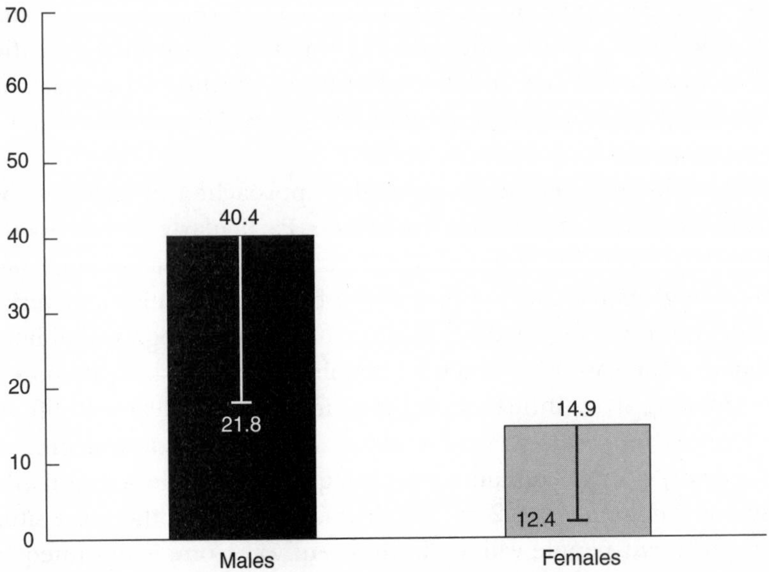

Figure 7.1. Sex differences in actor-centered decision making. Males exhibit a more context-dependent response selection pattern on the Cognitive Bias Task. Females exhibit a more context-independent response selection pattern. [After Goldberg et al. (1994). © 1994 by the Massachusetts Institute of Technology. Reprinted with permission.]

homogeneous mass, ignoring the self-evident truth apparent to every man and woman in the street: that males and females are different. But we are finding out increasingly that one ignores gender differences in cognition at one's own peril. Early work on cognitive gender differences focused on specific cognitive skills, on who is better in what. This inquiry focused on what we call here *veridical* decision making. Some of the most quoted research suggests, for instance, that males are better at mathematics and spatial relationships, and females are better at languages. But very little, if anything, has been said about gender differences in general cognitive styles. In particular, next to nothing has been said in the cognitive literature about gender differences in the general approach to decision making, about what we call here *adaptive* decision making. Our work with CBT is among the first such accounts.

Could the gender differences observed in our esoteric experiment correspond to some real-life traits? Common sense suggests that they could. Imagine two approaches to personal finances. Jane

Blane and Joe Blow are self-employed consultants whose incomes fluctuate from month to month. Jane Blane practices a context-independent approach to life. She always saves 5% of her income, never buys clothes costing more than $500 per item, and always takes her vacation in August. By contrast, Joe Blow's approach to life is context-dependent. When his monthly income is below $5000 he saves nothing, when it is between $5000 and $7000 he saves 5%, and he saves 10% when his monthly income exceeds $7000. He tends not to buy clothes costing more than $500, except when his monthly income is particularly high. He takes a vacation whenever his workload permits. This is just an example, but it models basic lifelong individual differences in actor-centered decision making.

In a very broad sense, the context-independent strategy can be thought of as a "universal default strategy." It represents an attempt by the organism to formulate all-purpose "best" responses averaged, in some sense, across all the possible life situations. The organism will accumulate a repertoire of such responses as a concise sum total of lifelong experiences. The "all-purpose" repertoire will be updated with new experiences, but very slowly and gradually, since it is the conservator of the individual's "universal wisdom."

The problem with such a strategy is that real-life situations are often so different from one another that any attempt at "averaging" becomes meaningless. In statistics, drawing a mean value across exemplars makes sense only if all the exemplars represent the same population. If the exemplars are drawn from different populations, then the mean will be misleading. Nonetheless, such a "default" strategy may be your best bet when you are faced with a totally novel situation, for which you have no specific experience or knowledge.

By contrast, a context-dependent strategy reflects an attempt to capture the unique, or at least specific, properties of the situation at hand and to "custom tailor" the organism's response. Having encountered a new situation, the organism attempts to recognize it as a familiar pattern representing a familiar *narrow class* of situation, a "known quantity." This accomplished, the organism applies the specific experience of dealing with such familiar situations. But faced with a radically new situation, the organism's attempt at pattern recognition will fail. In that case, an organism guided by a context-dependent strategy, a no-default option, will attempt to capture the unique properties of the situation at hand right away, even though the available information may be woefully insufficient. This will produce a "bouncy" behavior with precipitous changes at every transition to a new situation.

The optimal decision-making strategy is probably achieved through a dynamic balance between the context-dependent and context-independent approaches. Indeed, very few people adhere to one or the other strategy in its pure form; most people are able to switch between them at will, or to adopt mixed strategies, depending on the situation. But in subtle ways individuals tend to gravitate toward one or the other approach to life. Likewise, our research shows that females as a group have a subtle preference toward context-independence and males toward context-dependence.

Neither strategy is better than the other in an absolute sense. Their relative advantages depend on how stationary the environment is. In a relatively stationary environment a context-independent approach to decision making is probably the sounder one. In a highly unstable environment a context-dependent approach is preferable. The choice of strategy also depends on how good a grasp the individual in question has on the specific situations at hand. If his or her grasp on the specific situations at hand is good, then a context-dependent strategy is probably better. But if an individual's grasp on the specific situations is shaky because the individual lacks familiarity with the situation or because the situation is inherently complex, then it may be more prudent to rely on a compact set of tried and true default principles.

Evolution seems to value both decision-making strategies, and both are represented in our species. Do they work better synergistically than either one by itself? How do they complement each other? Which one is better suited for which type of cognitive challenges? What evolutionary pressures resulted in their slight divergence by sex? Do the two decision-making strategies adaptively suit the distinct male and female roles in our success as a species? Do these differences correspond to the different roles played by females and males at early stages of human evolution? Are the gender differences in decision-making styles biologically or culturally determined to begin with? Are these differences found in other primates? Or are they possibly even found in most mammalian species? Are people born with them, or do boys and girls diverge in their decision-making styles only as they approach sexual maturity? Does the decision-making style change in females with menopause? Do the gender differences in decision-making styles recede as the societal roles of males and females continue to converge? These fascinating questions await their answers through future research.

Research into cognitive gender differences, although increasingly prominent, is sometimes assaulted when a statement of gender *difference* is militantly misconstrued as a statement of gender *inferiority*. I was once a target of such misguided political correctness while giving a guest lecture at a prominent medical center in New York City in the mid-1990s. A young postdoctoral fellow interrupted my presentation and stridently accused me of male chauvinism as I was presenting the findings described in this chapter. I responded by saying that not having been particularly concerned about political correctness in my old country, the Soviet Union, where the consequences of political "incorrectness" could be quite dire, I saw no reason to worry about it in the United States, where the worst that could happen was wasting my time on a stupid argument. To their credit, the audience of doctors and medical students reacted with a round of applause.

It may be interesting to create a taxonomy of activities which lend themselves better to context-dependent and to context-independent decision making. To a degree, this can be accomplished empirically. But the distinction between the context-dependent and context-independent strategies also lends itself to relatively straightforward computational modeling with neural nets and other methods. In addition to modeling individual organisms, a collective behavior of such organisms can be examined, when some of them are "context-dependent" and some are "context-independent." Furthermore, the relative prevalence of these two decision-making biases can be varied in different environments. By examining such group behaviors of neural nets, it may be possible to begin to understand the adaptive value of having different decision-making strategies combined in a population. In the long run, such theoretical computational models may provide particularly important insights into the individual differences and the adaptive value of having several decision-making types represented in society.

Frontal Lobes, Hemispheres, and Cognitive Styles

What are the brain mechanisms of different cognitive styles? Do different decision-making strategies depend on different parts of the brain? Are these mechanisms different in males and females? Decision-making styles seem to depend on the frontal lobes. They also exhibit sex differences and are lateralized. This brings us to the issue of the lateralization of frontal lobe functions.

Hemispheric specialization has always been a central topic in neuropsychology. However, the frontal lobes have traditionally been on the periphery of such inquiry, an afterthought. This was an understandable consequence of the prevailing belief that the functional differences between the two hemispheres revolved around the "verbal–visuospatial" distinction. Since the prefrontal cortex has not been traditionally regarded as the "seat" of either language or visual–spatial processes, it was not regarded particularly pertinent to this distinction.

But this flies in the face of common sense, if we believe that brain structure and brain biochemistry have more than a passing relationship to brain function. The frontal lobes exhibit morphological gender differences and asymmetries, which humans share with several nonhuman species. The protrusion of the right frontal pole over the left frontal pole, known as the Yakovlevian torque (the other half of the torque includes a protrusion of the left occipital lobe over the right occipital lobe), is conspicuous in male humans and less pronounced in female humans. But it is present also in fossil man.[4] The cortical thickness of the left and right frontal lobes is similar in female humans but different in male humans (right thicker than left). Humans share the gender difference in frontal cortical thickness with several mammalian species. Humans also share the differences in left and right frontal cortical thickness in males with several other species.[5]

Biochemical differences found in the frontal lobes are also shared by humans with other species. Estrogen receptors are symmetrically distributed across the frontal lobes in female humans and asymmetrically distributed in male humans—and also in several nonhuman mammalian species.[6] Some of the major neurotransmitters also exhibit hemispheric asymmetry. Dopamine pathways tend to be more prevalent in the left than right frontal lobe, and noradrenergic pathways tend to be more prevalent in the right than left frontal lobe. This dual asymmetry is found in humans and in the monkey and the rat.[7]

With this background, it is highly probable that the frontal lobes are functionally different in males and females. It is also probable that the left and right frontal lobes are functionally different in males but less so in females. By the same token, it is highly *improbable* that these functional differences are restricted to the difference between language and nonverbal processes—for the simple reason that this distinction has no meaning in monkeys, rats, and such.

As before, my colleagues and I felt that we stood the best chance of cracking the problem by applying our nonveridical, actor-centered tasks. We chose for the study patients with isolated lesions in the left frontal lobe or the right frontal lobe, males and females. We first limited our study to right-handed patients. When we gave the Cognitive Bias Task to the patients, a rather striking picture emerged.

Males with a damaged right frontal lobe behaved in an extremely context-dependent manner and males with a damaged left frontal lobe behaved in an extremely context-independent manner. Neurologically intact normal controls were somewhere in the middle of the range. So it appears that in males the two frontal lobes make their choices in very different, in a way opposite, ways. In a normal brain these two decision-making strategies coexist in dynamic balance, with one or the other assuming the leading role depending on the situation. But this flexibility of decision making is lost in brain damage, and behavior deteriorates toward one or the other maladaptive extreme. In females the picture was entirely different. Both left and right frontal lesions produced extremely context-dependent behavior, whereas neurologically healthy normal females exhibited, as we already know, context-independent behavior.

Of course, the next logical step is to study normal subjects with functional neuroimaging, and this is what we are doing as of this writing. The expectation is that healthy right-handed males with the preference for context-dependent decision making will show a particular activation of the left prefrontal cortex while doing the task. By contrast, healthy right-handed males with the preference for context-independent decision making will show a particular activation of the right prefrontal cortex. In females a totally different picture can be expected. Healthy right-handed females with the preference toward context-independent decision making will show a particular activation of the prefrontal cortex bilaterally, and the females with the preference for context-dependent decision making will show a particular activation of the posterior cortex bilaterally.

Cognitive Styles and Brain Wiring

The male and female cognitive decision-making strategies are different, and so are the patterns of lateralization of their frontal lobe functions. It has been known for some time that structural, biochemical, and functional differences between the hemispheres are greater in males than in females.[8] So it should come as no surprise that the functional differences are greater between the two male frontal lobes than between the two female frontal lobes.

Among many possible ramifications of these differences, one is particularly interesting. It relates to the fact that various diseases of the brain afflict males and females at different rates. Schizophrenia,[9] Tourette's syndrome,[10] and attention deficit hyperactivity disorder[11] are all more common in men than in women. As we will find out later in this book, all three disorders are understood today as dysfunction of the frontal lobes, or of structures closely linked to the frontal lobes. Could it be that males are more vulnerable than females to any disorder affecting predominantly the frontal lobes? This could be due to the fact that the two female frontal lobes are functionally more alike and therefore each of them is more capable of taking over the functions of the other in the case of lateralized frontal lobe dysfunction. Indeed, a suggestion of lateralized, rather than completely bilateral, brain dysfunction is present in schizophrenia,[12] Tourette's syndrome,[13] and possibly even in attention deficit hyperactivity disorder.[14]

Does all this mean that female cortex is generally less functionally differentiated than male cortex? Traditionally this question was asked narrowly, only with respect to the cerebral hemispheres, and then the answer had to be yes. But recent research suggests that in certain respects the female cortex is *more* functionally differentiated than the male cortex. Our own work also pointed in this direction when we compared the effects of posterior (parietal and temporal) lesions on the response selection strategies.[15]

The effects of posterior (parietal and temporal) lesions in males and females on CBT performance were considerably less significant than the effects of frontal lesions. This was to be expected if actor-centered decision making is primarily under the control of the frontal lobes. Nonetheless, the effects of posterior brain lesions were also gender-dimorphic. In males the direction of posterior lesion effects was the same as the frontal lesion effects, albeit much weaker:

left-sided lesions made behavior more context-independent, and right-sided lesions made behavior more context-dependent. But in females the effects of posterior lesions were opposite to those of the frontal lesions: they made performance less context-dependent rather than more context-dependent.

Taken together, the male and female findings lead to a provocative conclusion. These findings challenge the established belief that the same pattern of functional cortical differentiation is present in both sexes, but expressed more strongly in males than in females. Our findings suggest that the difference is not merely in degree but in kind, that a qualitative difference is present. The female cortex is no less functionally differentiated than the male cortex—and no more. The two sexes emphasize different aspects of functional cortical differentiation. In the male brain the left–right differences are better articulated than in the female brain. But in the female brain the front–back differences are better articulated than in the male brain!

This conclusion is supported by earlier research studying the effects of lesions[16] and examining the patterns of regional cerebral blood flow[17] and functional magnetic resonance imaging (fMRI) activation in males and females.[18] When the task was to process verbal information, the co-activation of the frontal and posterior regions within the same hemisphere, the left, was seen in males. By contrast, in females the co-activation was symmetric ("homologous"), that is, co-activation of the two opposite hemispheres was recorded.

What could be the mechanism of these two alternative emphases in the male and female functional cortical organization? This question may be best dealt with if instead of functional *differentiation* we consider functional *integration*. The degree of functional integration as opposed to differentiation between brain structures depends, in turn, on the degree of interaction among them. The greater the interaction between two brain structures, the greater their functional integration. The more limited the interaction between these structures, the greater their functional differentiation.

With this reasoning in mind, let us consider what is known about the main connections within the brain. The corpus callosum is the structure that together with the anterior and posterior comissures, connects the two cortical hemispheres. Certain aspects of the corpus callosum are thicker in females than in males.[19] To the extent that we believe in a more or less direct relationship between structure and function (a tempting, albeit precarious proposition), this may account for greater functional interaction, hence greater functional integration and lesser functional differentiation, between the cortical hemispheres in females.

Next let us consider the main connecting structures between the front (anterior) and back (posterior) aspects of the *same* hemisphere, the longitudinal fasciculi and other long white matter bundles connecting distant cortical regions *within* a hemisphere. Recent studies have shown that these structures are somewhat larger in males than in females.[20] Following the logic of analysis that we adopted in this section, this may account for greater functional interaction, hence greater functional integration and lesser functional differentiation, between the frontal and posterior portions of a hemisphere in males.

A rather elegant, equitable picture of two complementary neuroanatomical connection emphases in males and females emerges, which may account for some of the fundamental cognitive differences between the two sexes. How exactly do these two patterns of connectivity affect cognition? Which pattern of connectivity is "better" for what cognitive task? What is the adaptive evolutionary value of having these two complementary patterns of neural organization represented within the species in roughly equal proportions (a teleological question that I keep asking at the risk of incurring the wrath of Stephen Jay Gould)?

These are all fascinating, and fundamental, questions. In trying to answer them it is tempting to capitalize on the relatively straightforward way in which the neuroanatomical gender differences described here lend themselves to formalization in a computational model. These questions are best answered, in my opinion, through experimentation with computational models, perhaps formal neural nets, comparing the emergent properties of enhanced connections *within* layers with the emergent properties of enhanced connections *between* layers in a bicameral model. Among the many challenges of cognitive neuroscience, those that allow natural (as opposed to contrived) theoretical models are particularly attractive, since they help move the field of neuropsychology out of the purely empirical domain into the domain of developed theoretical disciplines. The puzzle of cognitive differences between the sexes may prove to be among these challenges.

Rebels in Small Proportion: Handedness and Novelty Seeking

It would appear that novelty seeking should be the cardinal attribute of our restless species, but it is not. Humans tend to be conservative, gravitating toward the familiar. During my presentations for the general public I am always amused by how people want to hear what they already know and not what is truly novel. Journalists, including those who occasionally interview me about the brain for various features in the lay press, have the same inclination.

In fact, it can be argued that monkeys tend to be attracted to novelty much more than humans are. In an experiment Mortimer Mishkin and Karl Pribram conducted in the 1950s a monkey had to choose between an object identical to one previously shown and a different object.[21] The monkey saw an object. Then the monkey saw another object, which was either identical to the baited object or different from it. Two conditions were compared: when the identical (familiar) object was reinforced and when the different (novel) object was reinforced. On the whole, the monkeys learned to respond to novel stimuli faster than to the familiar ones, which suggests that they tend to be more attracted to the novel than to the familiar.

In a comparable situation, humans act in a very different manner. The preferences exhibited by our subjects on the Cognitive Bias Task (when they were asked to look at the target and make one of the two choices that they "liked the best") were very different from those of the monkeys. Humans almost invariably chose the items more similar to the target rather than the more different ones. This was true both for the right-handed healthy subjects and brain-damaged patients.

Such an emphasis on the familiar is understandable, since humans, at least adult humans, are guided by previously accumulated knowledge to a much larger extent than any other species. To put it in different terms, the ratio of de novo discovery to the previously accumulated body of knowledge is relatively low in adult humans compared to other species. This is because no other species has the mechanism of storing and transmitting the collective knowledge of the species accumulated over many generations in external cultural devices—books, films, and the like. Therefore, our bias toward the familiar serves an adaptive function. By contrast, the assimilation of previously accumulated knowledge in a monkey is limited to imitation of other monkeys' behavior. By and large, a young animal is embarked on a cognitive voyage, discovering its world on its own.

Human predisposition toward familiarity may change, as new knowledge accumulates at an exponential rate. A sociologist of science may someday devise a formula relating the amount of knowledge acquired within a generation to the amount of knowledge inherited from previous generations. The paradox is that this ratio changes in a nonmonotonic way. The ratio is high in nonhuman primates and probably during the prehistoric stages of human civilization; low through ancient history and dark middle ages; and picks up the speed through recent history, reaching exponential growth in modern times. The first peak of this ratio reflects an absence of effective cultural devices for information storage and transmission. By contrast, the second peak reflects the power of such devices, which permits an increasingly rapid accumulation of information. In human societies a low acquired-to-inherited knowledge ratio found in traditional cultures is associated with the cult of the elders as the repositories of accumulated wisdom. By contrast, a high acquired-to-inherited knowledge ratio found in modern societies is associated with the cult of the young as the vehicle of discovery and progress.

But a society cannot thrive on conservatism alone. For progress to occur, a mechanism must exist balancing conservatism and innovation. An excessively conservative society will be stagnant. A society too ready to give up established principles and concepts and rush headlong toward the new and untested ones will be dangerously flimsy and unstable. This delicate balance is maintained in every society through tacit conventions and explicit rules which determine how high the hurdle a new idea must clear to gain acceptance. Different societies set these hurdles at different levels for different situations. In science, for instance, the more radical a new idea, the higher the threshold for acceptance. An increasingly more rapid rate of knowledge accumulation through history is accompanied by the society's increasing willingness to revise the prevailing established assumptions. Yet it can be argued that even modern societies put a premium on preservation over modification.

Is there a mechanism operating at the biological, possibly genetic, level that regulates the balance between conservatism and innovation in human population? Merely phrasing a question in these terms has an outlandish, provocative ring. Yet our work has not only led me to suspect that such a mechanism exists, it even suggests what it may be.

I mentioned earlier that the overwhelming majority of our subjects showed preference for similarity on the Cognitive Bias Task—as long as they were right-handed. Among the left-handers the response pattern was distinctly different and many of them exhibited a preference for the choice which *differed* from the target rather than resembled it.[22] This was particularly true for the left-handed males. To the extent that our experiment elicits the preference toward the familiar versus the novel, it appears that left-handers, particularly left-handed males, are the novelty seekers.

Folkloric claims about the high prevalence of left-handedness among creative individuals have been around for many years. I have heard them repeated in different cultures on both sides of the Atlantic and have always dismissed them as gratuitous—until our own findings. Now I cannot help but entertain the intriguing possibility that different types of handedness may be associated with different biases toward the routine versus novel.

Handedness is not unique to humans. In many simian species, both apes and monkeys, one hand plays the leading role and the other hand plays a subordinate role consistently throughout the animal's lifetime.[23] The difference between us and them is that in simians no consistent preference is exhibited *within the population* and the handedness split across the members of the species is roughly even. In humans, on the other hand, approximately 90% of the population exhibits various degrees of right-handedness, and only about 10% gravitates toward left-handedness.[24] Among all the species exhibiting *individual* handedness, humans are the species that exhibits the most strong and consistent *population* trend in handedness.

Numerous prior attempts to find cognitive correlates of handedness basically failed.[25] What sets our study apart from most of the earlier research is our emphasis on actor-centered, rather than veridical, aspects of decision making. We are looking at cognitive *styles* rather than cognitive *abilities.* Once the question is phrased in this manner, an intriguing possibility emerges: left-handers are neither like right-handers nor are they the neuropsychological inverses of the right-handers, but they represent a distinctly different cognitive style.

If handedness is correlated with familiarity as opposed to novelty bias, then the roughly 9:1 ratio of right-handers to left-handers in the human population merits further examination. Could it be that this ratio reflects adaptive balance between conservation and innovation tendencies in the population, and that the population handedness bias serves as the mechanism to control this balance? Then left-handers are the innovation seekers, cultural rebels whose presence is necessary for societal ferment, but their proportion is best kept relatively low, lest society lose its broad cultural mooring.

To be viable, such a mechanism would have to allow some variation to regulate the conservation-to-innovation ratio in an adaptive manner. We do not know, how variable the "true" biological handedness ratio is in different cultures at different historical stages. We do know however, that cultural–anthropological factors affect this ratio in many societies. On the whole it seems that traditional societies, committed to the preservation of tradition more than innovation, tend to ostracize left-handedness and enforce right-handedness. Educational doctrines based on this tradition, perceived as misguided by modern Western society, persisted in most European and Asian societies well into the second half of twentieth century and continue to persist in many cultures even now. Born and schooled in eastern Europe, I am myself a product of this educational atavism and a converted lefthander. By contrast, the more dynamic North American society—less affected by cultural "baggage"—has been less bent on policing handedness, thus allowing a greater proportion of left-handers. While the enforced left- to right-handedness switch is very unlikely to change the underlying neurobiology and cognitive styles in any real sense, the policing of handedness may have been the traditional societies' naive reaction to the observations that iconoclastic behavior is often associated with left-handedness.

An even broader question can be asked. Is it possible that in other, nonhuman, primates handedness serves as a mechanism for regulating the conservation-versus-innovation population balance? Let's return to Mishkin's experiment. Could it be that in his sample the familiarity-seeking monkeys were right-handed, and the novelty-seeking monkeys were left-handed? Unfortunately, no handedness data are available.[26]

What are the mechanisms relating handedness to the conservation–innovation bias? In our earlier discussion we linked the left hemisphere with cognitive routines and the right hemisphere with cognitive novelty. Well then, by virtue of the contralaterality of motor control, right-handedness tends to preferentially engage the left hemisphere and left-handedness tends to preferentially engage the right hemisphere. This reasoning implies that the roles of the two hemispheres with respect to the novelty–routinization distinction are unchanged in right-handers and left-handers. However, our own research using actor-centered cognitive tasks has shown that the functional roles of the two frontal lobes are reversed in left-handers compared to right-handers.[27] This further highlights the complex relationship between handedness and hemispheric specialization. It could be, for instance, that certain aspects of hemispheric specialization are reversed in left-handers, while certain others remain unchanged.

Another possibility is prompted by the studies relating personality traits to brain biochemistry. People conspicuous in their predilection to risk taking seem to have an exceptionally high representation of a certain type of dopamine receptors.[28] Dopamine, of course, is a neurotransmitter particularly closely linked to the frontal lobes. Is it possible that this particular receptor type, an allele of D4 receptors, is particularly common among the left-handers? Is it particularly common among the people exhibiting novelty seeking on cognitive tasks such as the Cognitive Bias Task?

Until these questions are rigorously answered, the thesis developed in this chapter will remain speculative. Still, the intriguing possibility exists that the left-handers in our midst represent the restless, creative, novelty-seeking ferment in history—a catalyst indispensable for progress, yet best kept in check, lest it upset our societal apple cart.

Whatever the underlying neurobiology, on a phenomenal level we know that some people are better at innovation and others at following routines. Indeed, these different gifts are often incompatible. Visionaries who develop new trends in science, culture, or business often fail at implementing their own ideas in a sustained and systematic way; and other people, incapable of developing new trends but necessary to sustain them, have to take over to make things happen. Does this mean that trail-blazing visionaries have a particularly well-developed right hemisphere and cautious conventional types have a more developed left hemisphere? This is a fascinating proposition for the neuropsychology of individual differences to examine.

Like creativity, mental illness and neurodevelopmental disorders have also been linked to left-handedness. Schizophrenia, autism, dyslexia, attention deficit disorder are all characterized by an unusually high proportion of left-handers. While many cases of left-handedness are "pathological" (acquired due to early brain damage),[29] many others are hereditary, genetically determined. The parallels between creativity and madness have fascinated both scientists and poets. Particularly interesting are cases of fluid borders, of geniuses gone mad, like van Gogh and Nijinsky. Both genius and madness are deviations from the statistical norm. The romantic view holds that creative insights too far ahead of their time are often denounced by contemporaries as madness. The cynical view suggests that some of the more enduring cultural beliefs were a result of psychosis. Although the relationship between creativity and mental illness is well outside the scope of this book, their shared relationship to left-handedness is highly provocative.

Executive Talents: The S Factor and the Theory of Mind

Human brains are as variable in their individual features as any other part of the body. Weight, relative sizes of different lobes, the articulation of gyri and sulci—all are highly variable. Although the cognitive neuroscience of individual differences has yet to come together, it makes intuitive sense that the individual cognitive traits and talents have something to do with the individual variation in brain organization. Notably, the individual variation of human brain morphology is particularly pronounced in the frontal lobes.[30]

We tend to define people by their talents and shortcomings. Someone is musically gifted but has no spatial sense; someone else has a way with words but has a deaf ear. Such descriptions capture the person's special traits but not the person's essence. But when we call someone "smart" or "shrewd" and someone else "dumb" or "obtuse," we are no longer talking about narrow special traits. We are alluding to something both more elusive and more profound. We come much closer to defining the person's essence, to defining the person himself, rather than the person's attributes. Being "smart" (or "dumb") is not an attribute of you; it *is* you. Peculiarly, a certain degree of independence exists between this global dimension of human mind and the more narrow special traits. An individual may be devoid of any special talents, musical, literary, or athletic, yet be considered by others to be very "smart." The opposite is also possible, when a uniquely gifted individual is nonetheless perceived as "dumb." At the risk of committing cultural sacrilege, I will suggest that, based on biographic accounts, Mozart was probably somewhat a "dumb" genius. Lack of everyday wisdom could probably also be imputed in the case of one of my intellectual heroes, Alan Turing. Of course, the examples of the opposite, the "ordinary smart," are numerous and, by definition, anonymous. Many readers of this book will probably qualify.

But what do we mean by the terms "shrewd" and "obtuse"? And what are the brain structures whose individual variations determine these global traits? This question is directly related to the search for general intelligence—the "G factor"—and for measures of it, which are outside the scope of this book. The issue remains a matter of heated scientific debate. The last two decades have witnessed a departure from the notion of a single *G* factor in favor of "multiple intelligences." Introduced by Gardner[31] and Goleman,[32] these domain-specific "intelligences" broadly correspond to the cognitive variables systematically studied by cognitive neuroscientists and tested by clinical neuropsychologists and known to be dissociable in both neurological health and neurological illness.

Regardless of how the cognitive construct of general intelligence is defined, I am not aware of the existence of any distinct, single brain characteristic shown to account for such a *G* factor. The few available studies of genius brains failed to turn up compelling findings, and some of them are outright counterintuitive (which goes to show how flawed our intuitions are on the subject). For example, the brain of author Anatole France was known for its small size.[33] Einstein's brain reveals a peculiar lack of differentiation between the temporal and parietal lobes, as if a portion of the temporal lobe was "appropriated" by the parietal lobe.[34] This may possibly account for his self-reported preference for visualization over formalisms in developing his ideas (as well as for his reported dyslexia). But unless we believe in a homunculus inhabiting the general region of the angular/supramarginal gyrus, the finding is too local, too regional to account for an all-encompassing *G*. This leads us to the conclusion that many forms of "genius" reflect local properties of the mind (and by inference, of the brain) and may have little to do with our intuitive sense of "being smart" as a global, central, defining personal attribute. The local nature of genius is suggested by the biographic accounts of Mozart and Turing. Based on what we know of their lives, neither would have been regarded as "smart" by most people.

But what about the *S* factor (*S* for "smart")? I believe that, unlike the *G* factor, the *S* factor does exist. In this, I enjoy the tacit support of scores of ordinary people totally oblivious to *G* but acutely sensitive to *S*. Lay people, unencumbered by any particular psychological preconceptions but endowed with common sense, are amazingly confident, effortlessly and consistently judging who is smart—and who is not. What are they responding to in fellow human beings? What is the basis of their intuition? I have always thought this question worth asking but have been unable to find an answer in the literature. The underpinnings of everyday perception of intelligence are a fascinating subject on the interface of neuropsychology and social psychology.

The study that I envision should be as naturalistic as possible. Suppose you assemble a panel of lay "judges" unencumbered by any psychological preconceptions and unconstrained by excessive instructions from the researcher. Suppose, further, you recruit a sample of equally lay subjects. The judges have to rate the subjects on a ten-point scale of "smartness," based on a sample of live one-on-one freewheeling one-hour-long interaction or (less desirable) on a prerecorded tape of the subjects interacting with someone else or among themselves. The situation (live or taped) should be as naturalistic and unconstrained as possible. After the experiment all the subjects are put through an extensive battery of neuropsychological tests. What are your predictions? Do you expect the *S* ratings to be culture-dependent or culture-invariant?

I predict that the judges' ratings, or at least rankings, of the subjects would be highly consistent. Although cultural and professional factors undoubtedly play a role in judging "smartness," I believe that fundamental cultural invariants of "smartness" exist which are perceived similarly in every society, just as they have been suggested to exist for physical beauty. I predict further that of all the neuropsychological tests, the "smartness" ratings would be best correlated with the tests of executive functions. In the "multiple intelligence" scheme of things, it is the executive intelligence that we intuitively recognize as "being smart," the *S* factor. And of all the aspects of intelligence, the *S* factor—the "executive talent"—shapes our perception of a person as a persona, and not just as a carrier of a certain cognitive trait.

But every scale has its range defined by two extreme points. Therefore, rating people on the *S* factor is tantamount to rating them on a *D* factor (*D* for "dumb"). This turns the proposed experiment into a highly inflammatory enterprise, which may never see the light of day in our correctness-preoccupied culture. That would be a shame.

To a large extent, the trait in question refers to our ability to form the insight into other people and to anticipate their behavior, motives, and intentions. Given the communal nature of our lives, this ability is of paramount importance to our success in the broadest possible sense. Whether you want to cooperate with someone's intentions or thwart them (and particularly in the latter case), you must first understand and anticipate the other person's intentions.

In the earlier description of the essential executive functions I emphasized their sequential, planning, temporal ordering aspect. Now imagine that you have to plan and sequentially organize *your* actions in coordination with a group of other individuals and institutions engaged in the planning and sequential organization of *their* actions. Your relationship with these other individuals and institutions may be cooperative, adversarial, or both. Furthermore, the nature of this relationship may change over time. To succeed in this interaction, you must not only be able to have an action plan of your own, but you must also have an insight into the nature of the other fellow's plan. You must not only be able to foresee the consequences of your own actions, but you must also foresee the consequences of the other fellow's actions. To do that, you must have the capacity to form an internal representation of the other person's mental life or to use the high language of cognitive neuropsychology to form the "theory of mind" of the other person. Your own actions will then be chosen under the influence of your theory of the next fellow's mind formulated in your own mind. And the next fellow presumably will have a theory of *your* mind formulated in *his* head. The relative success of each of you will largely depend on the accuracy and degree of precision of your relative abilities to form the internal representation of the other. This makes the executive processes required for success in an interactive social (or rather *societal*) environment much more complex than the executive processes required in a solitary situation, such as solving a puzzle. This is true for competitive, cooperative, or mixed interactive situations.

Chess or checkers represents a formalized, highly distilled example of such "social" executive functions. The activities of business, political, or military leaders are also fundamentally based on their abilities to form the "theory of mind" of their opposite number, or very often their opposite numbers. In all such environments the essential questions are "What will he do next?" and "What should I do if he does this?" In my own experience, the game I had to play against the institutions of the state to extricate myself from the Soviet Union was the most extreme and demanding instance of a real-life high-stake chess game I have ever encountered. My capacity for insight into, and anticipation of, the other side's moves and intentions made all the difference between success and failure of my audacious enterprise.

The capacity for insight into other people's mental states is fundamental to social interactions. It finds very few prototypes in the animal world, if any. One of the most refined forms this capacity may take is deception, since deception requires manipulating the adversary into acquiring certain mental states, which the deceiver can then exploit. Frith and Frith argue that even apes lack this ability to any appreciable degree and that it is a uniquely human attribute.[35] The ironic corollary of this conclusion is that just as developed social interactions are uniquely human, so is sociopathy.

Someone with an insight into other people's minds is intuitively perceived as "smart" or "shrewd," and someone without this ability as "dumb" or "obtuse." We use these descriptions to capture the individual's cognitive essence as opposed to his narrow cognitive traits. While it may be possible to respect a "dumb" person's special gift, we find it very difficult to respect the person as an individual. And based on everything we know about the brain, this elusive but fundamental ability rests with the frontal lobes. In a number of studies normal subjects were asked to imagine the mental states of other people while their brains were being scanned with PET or fMRI. Invariably, particular activation was found in the medial and lateral inferior prefrontal cortex.[36]

We encounter enhanced capacity for insight into other people's inner worlds in successful corporate, political, and military leaders. But just as often, or more, we encounter this capacity diminished. Poor ability to form the theory of mind may be an expression of the normal variability in frontal lobe function without necessarily implying outright frontal lobe pathology, just as most everyday instances of inarticulate language do not imply outright damage to the temporal lobe.

As a clinician, I encounter this "benign" nonpathological diminution of the ability to form a theory of mind and presumably a subtle functional weakness of the frontal lobes quite frequently. I used to find it annoying but have come to enjoy it as a cognitive voyeur of sorts and a casual student of the individual variation of frontal lobe function in everyday life.

A patient walks into my office and I begin to inquire into the circumstances of his car accident. The response goes roughly as follows. "Last night I opened the fridge and saw that we are running out of milk. My wife always has cereal for breakfast and how is she going to have it without milk! So the next morning I had to go to the grocery to buy some milk. We have three groceries in the neighborhood but I always buy from Joe because he is a nice guy and we served in the Navy together. So I get into my green station wagon, but then it occurred to me that I need to go the bank first . . ." and on and on, until, with any luck, we get to the street intersection where the collision happened.

My good patient clearly failed to form an accurate theory of my mind, or else he would have spared me (and himself) all the details which have no relevance whatsoever to anything I need to know about his problem as a neuropsychologist. Is it an expression of the good man's frontal lobe damage suffered in the accident? I doubt it. The odds are that he has always been like that: a bit, well . . . "dumb." He is allowed: we recognize individual differences in everything and respect the normal curve. Besides, it turns out that my patient is an excellent amateur musician and I am not—individual differences again.

But here is a case of a much more extreme incapacity to form the theory of my mind, which forces me to conclude the presence of frank frontal lobe pathology. A man in his early forties was referred for a neuropsychological evaluation. He was suffering from a mysterious neurodegenerative disease, probably hereditary, unnamed, and malignant. He strode vigorously into my office, neatly dressed and well put together, without any discernible stigmata of a neurological patient. I put him through my standard history-taking interview: age, education, marital status, handedness. His responses were to the point, in well-formed language.

Then I asked about his favorite pastimes. "Movies!"—came the response with the exhilaration of an adolescent reliving his first trip to Disneyland. And before I could put in a word or ask my next question, a rapid-fire account of all the recently seen movies came out, one after another after another, with colorful detail, delivered in an excited language impatient to get it all out at once. My first impulse was to move things along, but then I decided to let them run their course and see what happens. The movie accounts kept coming out exuberantly an endlessly, dozens of them one after another. The man *was* into movies and has watched them *all*—and now I, his doctor, was being made privy to this unforgettable and joyful personal experience! The movie plots kept spilling out for about 40 minutes and would have continued to spill out, had I not interrupted my patient finally and moved things along.

The "movie man" is etched in my memory as a case of a patient without a clue about his doctor's informational needs. This was an order-of-magnitude more profound deficit in the patient's ability to form the theory of my mind than the earlier case of the milk-fetching car accident victim, and I strongly suspected the presence of frontal lobe damage. Indeed, the results of the subsequent neuropsychological testing were suggestive of particularly severe frontal lobe dysfunction. My patient's inability to monitor and control his own output is common in frontal lobe disease and is often considered one of its central features. As we will see in the cases of the injured student Vladimir and the horse-riding accident victim Kevin, it may take many forms. This consequence of frontal lobe dysfunction is particularly damaging to the individual's societal interactions both in overtly clinical forms and in more subtle relatively benign everyday forms.

Clearly, the ability to form an internal representation of a different person's mind is linked to another fundamental cognitive ability: the concept of *mental self and mental self–nonself differentiation.* The sense of self is fundamental to our mental life and it would appear that no complex cognition can exist without it. Yet scientific evidence suggests that the sense of self emerges late in evolution and is linked to the development of the frontal lobes.

Experimental studies of the evolution of the "self" concept use the method of self–nonself (or self–other) differentiation.[37] Suppose you put an animal in front of a mirror. Will it relate to its own image as to self or as to a different animal? Dogs relate to their own image as they would to a different animal. They bark, growl, and engage in dominance displays. Only great apes and to a lesser extent monkeys relate to their mirror image as their own self.[38] They use the mirror as an opportunity to groom hard-to-reach body parts and to erase marks painted on their foreheads by experimenters.

From these humble evolutionary beginnings, we humans have developed elaborate mental machinery for representing our own internal states. And again, the prefrontal cortex is implicated. When subjects are asked to focus on their own mental states, as opposed to external reality, medial prefrontal cortex lights up.[39] Both the internal representation of one's own mental states and the internal representations of the mental states of others rely on the frontal lobes. And so the complex, coordinated neural computations integrate and interweave the mental representations of "self" and "others." Truly, the prefrontal cortex is the closest there is to the neural substrate of social being.

That the capacity for self–nonself differentiation should depend on the frontal lobes comes as no surprise. As we have established before, the prefrontal cortex is the only part of the brain, and certainly of the neocortex, where information about the organism's internal environment converges with the information about the world outside. The prefrontal cortex is the only part of the brain with the neural machinery capable of integrating the two sources of data.

But how capable is it? How precisely does the emergence of this ability parallel the development of the frontal lobes? How closely does the development of this cognitive capability follow the emergence of its putative neural substrate? Is the development of self–nonself differentiation solely a function of frontal lobe emergence in evolution, or did it also require the emergence of certain conceptual structures incrementally externalized in the culture? In *The Origins of Consciousness and the Breakdown of the Bicameral Brain* Julian Jaynes proposed that self-consciousness emerged rather late in human cultural evolution, possibly as late as in the second millennium B.C.E.[40]

I also suspect that many enduring cultural beliefs (which, as a scientist, I tend to regard as "supernatural"), including religious beliefs, are vestiges of early humans' inability to recognize their own internal representations of other people as part of "self" rather than of "nonself." Rich sensory images of other persons, and even one's own thought processes, would be interpreted as "spirits." A rich sensory memory of a deceased tribesman would be interpreted as the tribesman's "ghost" or as evidence of the tribesman's "life after death." According to this scenario, some of the more literal religious and magical beliefs, which persisted for millennia, are vestiges of early humans' inability to distinguish between one's own memories of other people (internal representations, parts of "self") and those actual people themselves ("nonselves," others). This may have been precisely what Jaynes[41] refers to as the "hallucinatory experiences" of ancient humans. A careful cross-cultural investigation of cognitive self–nonself differentiation involving the few remaining relatively "primitive" cultures (e.g., Indian tribes of the Amazon, and Papua-New Guinea and Irian Jaya highlanders) could be particularly illuminating in this regard.

According to Jaynes, the self–nonself confusion was not confined to prehistoric times. It extended well into the early history populated by individuals we assume to be neurobiologically "modern." If this is so, then one of two possibilities (or a combination of the two) must be considered. First, the biological evolution of the frontal lobes is not in and of itself sufficient for the completion of cognitive self–nonself differentiation and that some additional, cumulative cultural effect is required, as Jaynes suggests. Or second, the biological evolution of the frontal lobes extended later into history than our established evolutionary assumptions would have it. The humanization of the great ape may have taken even longer than we thought.

8

When the Leader Is Wounded

The Fragile Frontal Lobes

The definition of disease changes over time. Classic neuropsychology was concerned with the effects of brain lesions (bullet wounds, strokes, and tumors) on cognition. This was the knowledge base on which our understanding of brain function was built. Gradually, the scope of neuropsychology has expanded, and today there are more neuropsychologists employed in psychiatric and geriatric settings than on traditional neurology services.

The expansion of neuropsychology reflects the expansion of the definition of brain disease. This, in turn, is a consequence of our society becoming more enlightened, more affluent, and, our occasional misgivings notwithstanding, on the whole more humane. In the old days, it was considered normal that by a certain age people would start "losing their marbles." Today we know that this is not part of normal aging, but rather a consequence of distinct brain disorders, such as Alzheimer's disease. In the old days, a poor learner was scolded by his parents, and an unruly pupil was flogged. Today we know about learning disabilities and attention deficit disorder.

I recall my first faculty position in the United States in the late 1970s at one of the most prestigious Ivy League departments of psychiatry. Clinical conferences were replete with endless debates over whether a particular patient was "schizophrenic" or "organic," organic meaning suffering a dysfunction of the brain. The old Cartesian distinction between the body and the soul, which had fooled the general public for so many years, had permeated psychiatry as well.

Today we know that schizophrenia is organic, since both biochemical and structural abnormalities have been discovered in the patients' brains. This is also true for depression, obsessive-compulsive disorder, attention deficit disorder, Tourette's syndrome, and other conditions. The distinction between the "diseases of the brain" and "diseases of the soul" is becoming increasingly blurred. The ailments of the "soul" are understood increasingly as the diseases of the brain. "Descartes' error," to use Antonio Damasio's elegant phrase,[1] is finally being corrected.

As we continue to discover the neural basis of the diseases previously thought to be in the soul department, the extreme degree of frontal lobe involvement in virtually all of these conditions becomes increasingly apparent. This speaks to a particular biological vulnerability of the frontal lobes. Indeed, frontal lobe dysfunction often reflects more than direct damage to the frontal lobes.[2]

The frontal lobes seem to be the bottleneck, the point of convergence of the effects of damage virtually anywhere in the brain.[3] Considering the military analogy, this should not come as a surprise. Injury to the leader will disrupt the activities of many units in the field, producing remote effects. Equally, the functions of leadership will be disrupted if the lines of communication from the front to the leader are cut off.

Damage to the frontal lobes produces wide ripple effects through the whole brain. At the same time, damage anywhere in the brain sets off ripple effects interfering with frontal lobe function. This unique feature reflects the role of the frontal lobes as the "nerve center" of the nervous system with a singularly rich set of connections to and from other brain structures.

The unique sensitivity of the frontal lobes to brain disease can be demonstrated in a number of ways. Swedish neuroscientists Asa Lilja and Jarl Risberg studied the patterns of regional cerebral blood flow (rCBF) disruption caused by brain tumors.[4] To their surprise, they found the blood flow particularly disrupted in the frontal lobes regardless of tumor location. This was true even if the tumor itself was as far away from the frontal lobes as you could get without leaving the cranium, so to speak.

Scientists at the New York State Psychiatric Institute studied regional blood flow patterns in patients with depression.[5] Disruption of blood flow was most pronounced in the frontal lobes, despite the fact that serotonin (a major neurotransmitter whose deficiency is presumed to be responsible for depression) is ubiquitous in the brain, without showing any particular frontal lobe preponderance. In Sweden, Risberg studied the transient effects of electroconvulsive therapy (ECT) on regional cerebral blood flow.[6] Again, most disruption was found in the frontal lobes even though the electrodes through which the current was delivered to the brain were applied to the temporal lobes.

In another study conducted at the New York State Psychiatric Institute, healthy volunteers were given scopolamine, a chemical substance interfering with the action of acetylcholine, one of the main neurotransmitters in the brain.[7] Scopolamine was given to create an experimental simulation of memory disorders in Alzheimer's disease. (The rationale for the experiment was based on the assumption that cholinergic transmission is particularly affected in Alzheimer's disease.) Again, the greatest disruption of regional cerebral blood flow was observed in the frontal lobes—despite the fact that unlike some other neurotransmitters, acetylcholine is not exceptionally prevalent in the frontal lobes.

Working at the New York University Aging and Dementia Center my colleagues and I have shown that frontal lobes become dysfunctional at a very early stage of Alzheimer's type dementia.[8] This is expressed as an inability to make decisions in ambiguous situations. Given the ambiguous nature of most real-life situations, the loss of this ability is fraught with particularly devastating consequences.

But cognitive changes occur in normal aging as well. It is not uncommon for people in their sixties and seventies to notice that their memory is not quite as sharp as it used to be. What most people fail to realize is that the so-called normal age-related changes affect the functions of the frontal lobes as much as they affect memory.

To conclude, the frontal lobes are more vulnerable and are affected in a broader range of brain disorders, neurodevelopmental, neuropsychiatric, neurogeriatric, and so on, than any other part of the brain. The frontal lobes have an exceptionally low "functional breakdown threshold." This led me many years ago to conclude that frontal lobe dysfunction is to the brain disease what fever is to bacterial infection. It is both highly predictable and often nonspecific.[9] Hughlings Jackson understood this very well when he introduced his law of "evolution and dissolution."[10] According to this law, the phylogenetically youngest brain structures are the first to succumb to brain disease. But I believe that the frontal lobes' unique vulnerability is the price they pay for the exceptional richness of their connections. The "noise summation" effect, the aggregation of faulty signals which probably take place in the prefrontal cortex following diffuse brain damage, can be demonstrated computationally. In fact, I designed a mathematical demonstration of this effect in collaboration with Yelena Artemyeva at the University of Moscow in the late 1960s using John von Neumann's parallel low-reliability automata as the model. The clinical corollary of this conclusion is that frontal lobe dysfunction does not always signify a frontal lobe lesion. In fact, in most instances it probably does not. Instead, it is a remote effect of a diffuse, distributed, or distant lesion.

Frontal Lobe Syndromes

Consider the sequence of events required for every purposeful behavior. First, behavior must be initiated. Second, the objective must be identified, the goal of action formulated. Third, a plan of action must be forged according to the goal. Fourth, the means by which the plan can be accomplished must be selected in a proper temporal sequence. Fifth, the various steps of the plan must be executed in an appropriate order with a smooth transition from step to step. Finally, a comparison must be made between the objective and the outcome of the action: Does the outcome correspond to the objective? Is it "mission accomplished" or "mission failed"? If "failed," then by how much and in which aspect of the task? In a nutshell, these are the functions of the executive in charge of the workings of an organization. These are also the functions of the frontal lobes. This is why the frontal lobe functions are often called "executive functions."

The importance of executive functions can be best appreciated through the analysis of their disintegration following brain damage. A patient with damaged frontal lobes retains, at least to a certain degree, the ability to exercise most cognitive skills in isolation.[11] The basic abilities, such as reading, writing, simple computations, verbal expression, and movements, remain largely unimpaired. Deceptively, the patient will perform well on the psychological tests measuring these functions in isolation. However, any synthetic activity requiring the coordination of many cognitive skills into a coherent, goal-directed process will become severely impaired.

But even a cursory review of frontal lobe neuroanatomy suggests their tremendous complexity. This, in turn, suggests a functional diversity of each distinct part. And indeed, damage to different parts of the frontal lobes produces distinct, clinically rather different syndromes. The most common among them are the *dorsolateral* and *orbitofrontal* syndromes.[12]

In early neurological literature the dorsolateral syndrome was known as "pseudodepression." The name alludes to the similarity of some frontal lobe patients to depressed patients. In both conditions extreme inertia and inability to initiate behaviors is present, sometimes to a high degree. A patient with a severe dorsolateral frontal syndrome will lie passively in bed, not eating, drinking, or attending to any other needs. He will fail to respond readily to any attempt to engage him in any activity. He will look somewhat like a patient with severe depression. But the similarity ends here. A depressed patient has a sad mood and a sense of pervasive misery, but a dorsolateral frontal patient has a flat affect and sense of indifference. The patient with dorsolateral frontal lesion is neither sad nor happy; in a sense, he has no mood. No matter what happens to the patient, good things or bad things, this state of indifference will persist.

The indifference of dorsolateral frontal patients is sometimes so extreme that it reduces their response to pain. Most people have heard about frontal lobotomy, a neurosurgical procedure severing the connections between the frontal lobes and the rest of the brain.[13] Introduced in 1935 by a Portuguese physician, Egas Moniz,[14] frontal lobotomy had its heyday in the United States in the 1940s and 1950s and has since been discredited and largely abandoned. For better or worse, it was used most often to treat psychosis. It was also used, however, to treat intractable pain, a rare condition of extreme suffering unresponsive to medications.

Frontal lobotomy, or a related procedure called "cingulotomy," "cured" such patients, permanently or temporarily, from the subjective feeling of suffering, but not from the physical sensation of pain.[15] Bizarrely, they continued to report their sensation in terms virtually identical to those used before the surgery. But what was once the source of unbearable suffering was now met with utter indifference. The patients were no longer bothered by pain, despite its persistent presence.

Robert Iacono, a neurosurgeon from southern California, brought to my attention the case of a patient suffering from excruciating and debilitating rectal pain with depression, sleep disturbance, and morphine addiction. Following cingulotomy, the patient no longer initiated complaints about pain, even though she continued to complain about pain when asked. For the first time in many months she appeared relaxed. The family was astonished at her personality change from extremely demanding to eerily compliant. During the next few weeks the patient's sleep notably improved and she voiced considerably fewer spontaneous complaints. She also became highly suggestible.[16]

The observation is extremely interesting, since it informs us both about the frontal lobes and about the mechanisms of pain. The sensory experience alone is not sufficient to produce the subjective feeling of suffering. A higher-order interpretative process is required, which appears to be somehow linked to the frontal lobes. Recent functional neuroimaging studies have shown, for instance, that the expectation of pain activates the medial frontal lobe regions.[17] When the signal about the aversive sensory experience fails to reach the frontal lobes, the experience fails to cause the subjective, affective sense of suffering. Frontal lobotomy "cured" by producing the dorsolateral frontal lobe syndrome in the patient. As will be made clear by the following discussion, the price of such a cure is very high.

Drive and Newtonian Bodies: A Dorsolateral Case Study

Vladimir was a promising engineering student in Moscow in his mid-twenties. He was standing on the platform of the Moscow subway, the famous, bombastically imposing "metro," Stalin's great pyramid built with the labor of Gulag slaves. When the soccer ball Vladimir was tossing around fell on the rails, he jumped down to get it. He was hit by an approaching train, suffered severe head injury, and was rushed to the Bourdenko Institute of Neurosurgery, where I did my research at the time under Luria's supervision. I first encountered Vladimir two or three months after his injury. By that time Vladimir was medically stable, his life no longer in danger.

Vladimir was particularly interesting because, as a result of his injury, he had to undergo surgical resection of both frontal poles.

Luria was becoming increasingly interested in the frontal lobes and I, the youngest among his immediate entourage, was as yet unattached to any particular project. So the frontal lobes became my project and Vladimir became "my" patient. Conveniently, I was one of the few males on Luria's largely female staff and thus could be relied on to deal with Vladimir's clinical antics.

The career of every clinician is punctuated by a few formative cases. Vladimir was my first formative case. Unwittingly, through his tragedy, he introduced me to the rich phenomena of frontal lobe disease, triggered my interest in the frontal lobes, and so helped shape my career. We were roughly the same age, in our twenties, he a few years older.

Vladimir spent most of his time in bed staring blankly into space. He ignored most attempts to engage him in any kind of activity. Persistent attempts could provoke a trickle of profanities, and a particularly vigorous intruder ran the risk of being hit with a chamber pot. Occasionally attracted by something in his environment, Vladimir attempted to get out of bed, but the bed was surrounded with a protective net.

The nurses would call on me to help coax Vladimir out of bed to go for a medical procedure or to give him an injection (the surest way to encounter Vladimir's chamber pot). I reasoned with Vladimir in a casually profane, locker room–style banter, and it usually had a calming effect. A friendship of sorts developed between a brain-damaged student and a student of brain damage. As a result, I was able to engage Vladimir in all kinds of little bedside experiments with relative ease, despite his general inertia. He would follow my instructions in a detached, stone-faced, zombielike fashion.

To most of us the word "drive" connotes a certain personality trait, one particularly valued in our achievement-oriented society. We associate drive with accomplishment, competition, success, winning spirit. A person without a drive is perceived as a loser unworthy of respect, almost an anomaly in our competitive culture. To most people, drive is a highly desirable social trait, a virtual sine qua non.

Like most human traits, drive has a biological basis. The frontal lobes are central to the maintenance of drive. I like to compare patients with dorsolateral frontal lobe disease to bodies in Newtonian physics. To set in motion a body in classical Newtonian mechanics, an application of external force is required. Likewise, external force is required to terminate motion or to set it on a new course. In an odd way, patients with dorsolateral frontal damage behave like Newtonian objects. The most conspicuous feature of their behavior is an inability to initiate any behavior. Once engaged in a behavior, however, the patient is equally unable to terminate or change it on his own.

Vladimir's inertia, so striking in his everyday behavior (or lack thereof), could also be elicited experimentally. Asked to draw a cross, he would first ignore the instruction. I had to lift his hand with mine, place it on the page, and give it a little push, and only then would he start drawing. But having started, he could not stop and continued to draw little crosses until I took his hand in mine and lifted it off the page (Fig. 8.1). Such combined inertia of initiation and termination is seen in various disorders affecting the frontal lobes, including chronic schizophrenia.

When the task was to listen to a story and then recall it, Vladimir would start slowly and then carry on in a monotonous voice. He would go on and on and when asked to finish, he would say "Not yet." The never-ending monologue was an expression of "reverse inertia," an inability to terminate activity.

I asked Vladimir to listen to a simple children's story, "A Lion and a Mouse," and then recall it. The story goes as follows:

> A lion was asleep and a mouse was running around him making noises. The lion woke up, caught the mouse, and was about to eat him up, but then decided to show mercy and let the mouse go. A few days later, hunters caught the lion and tied him to a tree with ropes. The mouse learned about it, ran down, gnawed the ropes and set the lion free.

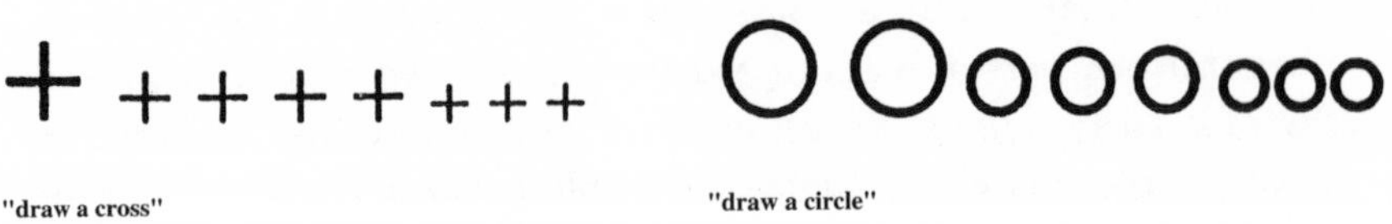

Figure 8.1. A frontal-lobe patient as a Newtonian body. A patient is asked to draw a cross. It takes a long time to entice him to do it, but then he is unable to terminate the process and keeps drawing crosses. Sometime later he is asked to draw a circle and the same cycle ensues. [Adapted from Goldberg and Costa (1985). Reprinted with permission.]

This is how Vladimir recalled the story:

> So the lion made friends with the mouse. The mouse was caught by the lion. He wanted to strangle him but then let him go. The mouse started dancing around him, singing songs, and was released. After that the mouse was accepted in his house by . . . lions, various animals. After that he was released, so to speak, he hadn't been captured, he was still free. But after that he was completely released and was walking free . . .

at this point I asked: "Are you finished?" But Vladimir said: "Not yet" and carried on:

> So, he was released by the lion completely, after the lion listened to him, and he was released to go to all the four directions. He didn't run away and remained to live in his cave. Then the lion caught him again, some time later . . . I don't remember it exactly. So he caught him and released him again. Now the mouse got out of there and went to his hangout, to his pad. The mouse goes on and on and talks about his pad. And there is another mouse there. So the mouse opens the door to this . . . what do you call it? Hi! Hi! How are you doing! OK, more or less. I am all set. Glad to see you. I have an apartment . . . and a house . . . and a room. The bigger mouse asks the smaller one: How are you doing? How is it coming along?

I say: "You better finish." But Vladimir again says: "Not yet!" and continues:

> So it was all right. I had a lot of friends. They often get together . . . but the friendship broke up, so tell him that I miss these brief get-togethers . . .

Vladimir continued his monologue until I turned off the tape-recorder and left.

Vladimir's inertia, both the inertia of initiation and the inertia of termination, was pervasive. It was evident both in his drawings and in his verbal output. The pervasive nature of inertia is typical in dorsolateral frontal lobe syndrome.

Vladimir's case was extreme. But following even mild head trauma, it is common for the patient to become indifferent and devoid of initiative and drive. The change may be subtle, and it is not always apparent to family members or even doctors that the change is neurological in nature, that it is a mild form of the frontal lobe syndrome. These symptoms are often called "personality change," but "personality" is not an extracranial attribute of a person, carried on our skin. Our personality is determined to a large extent by our neurobiology, and personality disorders, unlike skin disease, are caused by changes in the brain. The frontal lobes have more to do with our "personalities" than any other part of the brain, and frontal lobe damage produces profound personality change.

Subtle decrease of drive, initiative, and interest in the world around is also a common early sign of dementia. In the popular folklore early signs of dementia are associated with memory loss first and foremost. In reality, however, subtle frontal lobe dysfunction is as common.

Just how elusive frontal lobe symptoms can be for an uninitiated eye becomes clear from the example of Jane, a woman in her late fifties referred to me for a second opinion. A few years earlier Jane had developed tremors and was promptly referred to one of the best movement disorders clinics in town. The diagnosis of Parkinson's disease was promptly made and Jane was put on Sinemet, a dopamine-enhancing medication commonly used in these circumstances. But gradually a cognitive impairment became noticeable, affecting her memory, attention, and judgment. When her family members brought this to the doctors' attention, they were not particularly concerned and changed the Sinemet dosage. But contrary to their expectations, Jane's cognition did not improve. Quite the contrary, it continued to deteriorate. Then she lapsed into a psychotic episode, running up and down the block undressed, screaming that her neighbors were setting the building on fire. Other psychotic episodes followed, mostly with paranoid overtones. There was also some suggestion of hallucinations.

At this point, Jane's tremors were the least of the family's concerns, and they kept pleading with the doctors to do something about the cognitive impairment and psychosis. But the doctors just continued to adjust the Sinemet doses. They obviously assumed that the psychosis and the memory loss were the side effects of the medication. But there was no improvement and things were getting out of hand. Finally, the exasperated family decided to seek another opinion, as it happened, from me.

The history of Jane's illness was recounted to me by her husband, a lucid, educated, and caring man in his early sixties, a senior executive. The story had the telltale ring of Lewy bodies disease, a lesser-known dementia with a clinical course often actually more malignant than in Alzheimer's disease. Jane was taken off Sinemet and put on Cognex, a cholinergic enhancer, and a slight improvement was noted.

Becoming increasingly convinced that Jane indeed suffered from Lewy bodies disease, I decided to probe her husband a little more about the very early disease stage. As a result, a strikingly different clinical picture emerged. As it turned out, Jane's husband had left out a very significant feature of Jane's condition. At least a year prior to the first appearance of the tremors and possibly even earlier, a subtle change in Jane's personality had become increasingly apparent. Always vivacious and sociable, a great entertainer who put a lot of energy and gusto into her social life, Jane began to withdraw.

Uncharacteristically, she began to refuse to go out, preferring to stay at home. She stopped entertaining, saying that she had no energy or interest. Jane's husband had noticed the change and responded with a mixture of concern and annoyance. But it simply did not occur to this highly intelligent and devoted man that the changes in his wife's personality signaled a clinical disorder. Had this thought crossed his mind, the whole process of Jane's treatment would have taken a different course from the beginning. As it stands, it was obvious to me that Jane's "personality change" reflected the involvement of her frontal lobes at the earliest stage of the disease, well before the tremors or anything else.

Plans and the "Memories of the Future"

In 1985 David Ingvar, a Swedish psychiatrist and neuroscientist, coined a phrase both poetic and implausible: "Memory of the future."[18] What is a memory of the future? Memories are supposed to be about the past.

The confusion is resolved when we consider one of the most important functions of advanced organisms: making plans and then following the plans to guide behavior. Unlike primitive organisms, humans are active, rather than reactive, beings. The transition from mostly reactive to mostly proactive behavior is probably the central theme of the evolution of the nervous system. We are able to form goals, our visions of the future. Then we act according to our goals. But to guide our behavior in a sustained fashion, these mental images of the future must become the content of our memory; thus the memories of the future are formed.

We anticipate the future based on our past experiences and act according to our anticipations. The ability to organize behavior in time and to extrapolate in time is also the responsibility of the frontal lobes. Whether you have good foresight and planning ability or fly by the seat of your pants depends on how well your frontal lobes work. Patients with frontal lobe damage are notorious for their inability to plan and to anticipate the consequences of their actions. Damage to other parts of the brain does not seem to affect these abilities. One of the first signs of dementia, a subtle impairment of planning and foresight, is also present in other conditions, usually reflecting frontal lobe dysfunction.

A simple experiment illustrates Vladimir's severely impaired ability to follow plans. I asked Vladimir to listen to a story, "A Hen and Golden Eggs," and then recite it from memory. The story goes as follows:

> A man owned a hen that was laying golden eggs. The man was greedy and wanted to get more gold at once. He killed the hen and cut it open hoping to find a lot of gold inside, but there was none.

Vladimir repeated the story as follows:

> A man was living with a hen . . . or rather the man was the hen's owner. She was producing gold . . . The man . . . the owner wanted more gold at once . . . so he cut the hen into pieces but there was no gold . . . No gold at all . . . he cuts the hen more . . . no gold . . . the hen remains empty . . . So he searches again and again . . . No gold . . . he searches all around in all places . . . The search is going on with a tape-recorder . . . they are looking here and there, nothing new around. They leave the tape-recorder turned on, something is spinning there . . . what the hell are they recording there . . . some digits . . . 0, 2, 3, 0

> . . . so they are recording all these digits . . . not very many of them . . . that's why all the other digits were recorded . . . turned out to be not very many of them either . . . so, everything was recorded . . . [monologue continues][19]

The sheer length of Vladimir's monologue is out of proportion to the original story. This is his inability to terminate an activity—the inertia in reverse that we have already discussed. He also perseverates, as he continues to rehash the phrases and themes of the story. But at a certain point new content is introduced, a spinning tape-recorder. All of a sudden, Vladimir's story is a complete non sequitur: it is no longer about the golden eggs, but about a tape-recorder.

The explanation for this strange behavior lies in the environment. I am sitting in front of Vladimir with a portable tape-recorder in my lap, taping the very monologue that we are discussing here. Vladimir's task is to recall the story. The tape-recorder is completely incidental to this task. But its mere presence in the environment is sufficient to derail Vladimir's ability to follow the task at hand. Instead of being guided by the plan of action, Vladimir merely recites what he sees in front of him: the spinning and blinking of the tape-recorder. His train of thought is hopelessly lost and no longer bears any relation to the task at hand. He is unable to recapture the lost train of thought and continues to engage in his "field-dependent" digression.

Being at the mercy of incidental distractions and displaying an inability to follow plans are common features of frontal lobe disease. This is known as *field-dependent behavior.* A frontal lobe patient will drink from an empty cup, put on a jacket belonging to someone else, or scribble with a pencil on the table surface, merely because the cup, the jacket, and the pencil are there, even though these actions make no sense. This phenomenon was studied extensively by the French neurologist François Lhermitte, who called it "utilization behavior."[20]

I recall the indignation of the nurses on the university hospital neurology service where I used to consult many years ago. A few patients on the unit invariably kept wandering into the other patients' rooms, inciting the wrath of the nurses, who accused the patients of every conceivable malicious intent. The reality was much simpler and sadder. The wandering patients were entering through the doors just because the doors were there. They were patients with frontal lobe damage suffering from field-dependent behavior.

In the most extreme cases, field-dependent behavior takes the form of direct imitation, called "echolalia" (imitation of speech) or "echopraxia" (imitation of action). Instead of answering a question (an act requiring the formation of an internal plan) the patient merely repeats the question or incorporates the question into the answer. When asked "What is your name?" Vladimir would sometimes say: "What is my name Vladimir." Other patients imitate the doctor's actions: if I pick up a pen to write a chart note, the patient will pick up another pen and begin to scribble. Like other symptoms, echo behaviors may take subtle forms in naturalistic environments. On numerous occasions I would catch myself, in the middle of interviewing a patient, doing something entirely unrelated: scratching my nose or adjusting my glasses. The next thing I would notice is the patient engaging in the same unrelated act.

Field-dependent behavior is a complex phenomenon, which may take many forms. Sometimes field-dependent behavior is driven by external stimuli in the outside world, and sometimes it is driven by internal out-of-context associations. As we follow Vladimir's narrative, it takes a turn that finds no ready explanation in the external environment. Following the mention of the tape-recorder and of number 5 "spinning there," Vladimir begins to describe the route of city bus number 5 in downtown Moscow. This is also field-dependent behavior, but now the distractor is found not in the world outside, but among the internal associations in Vladimir's own memory. Thus the ability of a frontal lobe patient to stay mentally on course can be disrupted by both external and internal distractors.

Vladimir talks on and on in a monotonous, detached tone of voice. His tale spins by itself, through no apparent mental effort or intentional contribution on his part, one association or external stimulus leading to another. Finally I turn off the tape-recorder and begin to leave. Vladimir continues to ramble for a few more minutes and finally stops.

As noted earlier, Vladimir's ability to act according to an internal plan is severely impaired. But in many cases this deficit takes very subtle forms, not apparent through simple observation and requiring special tests to detect. One such test is known as the Stroop Test, after the name of its inventor.[21] Here the subject is asked to look at a list of color names printed in discordant colors (e.g., word "red" printed in blue or the other way around), and to name the colors, instead of reading the words.

What makes the Stroop Test so interesting? It requires that you contravene your immediate impulse. The impulse is to read the words; this is the natural tendency of every literate person on seeing written material. But the task is to name the colors. To successfully complete the task, you must follow the internal plan, the task, *against your natural, entrenched tendency.*

Most of us can exercise the ability to guide behavior by internal representation so effortlessly that we take it for granted. Bombarded by a myriad of incidental external stimuli and unrelated internal associations, we nonetheless stay on the "mental course" with ease, until the task is brought to successful conclusion. But trivial as it may appear, this ability arises relatively late in evolution.

The capacity to respond to external stimuli is the first attribute of a primitive brain. In an environment rich with events, however, such a primitive brain will be immediately overwhelmed by a plethora of random distractors. In a more complex brain, this will be balanced by a mechanism protecting the organism from the chaos of randomness and allowing it to stay on track in pursuing a particular behavior. Evolution of the brain is characterized by the slow, painstaking transition from a brain simply reacting to a brain capable of sustained, deliberate action.

Saying that life is full of distractions is so obvious it is almost cliché. However, the ability to stay on a course charted by an internal plan, a "memory of the future," arises quite late in evolution, as does the capacity for sustained attention. Their advent parallels the development of the frontal lobes.

Most of us have had encounters with a canine, or simply a dog. Suppose a dog is exploring an object when there is a distracting noise. This causes the dog to turn its head away from the object, toward the source of noise. Unless the object is food, the chances that the dog will go back to exploring the same object after the interruption are slim to nonexistent. This does not mean that the dog failed to form an internal representation of the object, since on subsequent encounters it will exhibit familiarity with the object. It does mean, however, that the mental representation fails to exert an effective control over canine behavior. One of the most prominent students of the frontal lobes, Patricia Goldman-Rakic of Yale University, refers to this "afrontal" behavior as "out of sight, out of mind."[22]

There were always dogs in our household when I was growing up, and I can generally anticipate and "understand" their behavior to the extent that a middle-aged Manhattan intellectual can. But nothing in my canine encounters prepared me for my first truly interactive experience with an ape, albeit a "lesser" ape. As we shall see, an ape's behavior is strikingly different from that of a canine in response to a distractor.

While on vacation in Phuket, an island off the coast of southern Thailand, a number of years ago, I befriended and was befriended by a young black male gibbon from Laos, a pet of the owners of a restaurant next to my hotel. For about a week, I spent a few hours with him every day. Every morning the gibbon rushed forth to shake hands. All limbs and a small body, he would then engage in a brief spiderlike dance, which, in my self-flattering way, I interpreted as an expression of joy at seeing me. But then, despite his proclivity for restless play, he would settle next to me and with extreme concentration would study the minute details of my clothes: a watchband, a button, a shoe, my glasses (which, in one of my unguarded moments, he took off my face and tried for lunch). He stared at the items intently and systematically shifted his gaze from one detail to another. When one day a bandage appeared around my index finger, the young gibbon studiously examined it. Despite his status of a lesser ape (in contrast to the bonobos, chimpanzees, gorillas, and orangutans, which are known as the great apes), the gibbon was capable of sustained attention.

Most remarkably, the gibbon invariably turned back to the object of his curiosity following a sudden distraction, say, a street noise. He would resume his exploration precisely where it had been interrupted, even when the interruption was more than a split second in length. The gibbon's actions were guided by an internal representation, which "bridged" his behavior between before and after the distraction. "Out of sight" was no longer "out of mind"! My neuroscientific preconceptions aside, as a past owner of several dogs and a lifelong dog lover, I can vouch that this behavior was utterly uncanine. Not surprisingly, the canine frontal lobes account for approximately 7% of the total cortex, whereas in the gibbon it is 11.5%.[23]

The interaction with the gibbon was so qualitatively different from, and so strikingly richer than, anything I had ever experienced with dogs, that I briefly entertained the idea of buying the gibbon and bringing him to New York to be my pet and companion. The restaurateurs were game and the price was being discussed. But in the end sanity prevailed and I returned to my fiftieth-floor midtown Manhattan apartment alone.

In humans the capacity for "staying on track" takes on an even more complex dimension. Not only can we stay on track in attending to *external* objects, but we can also stay on track with respect to our own thoughts, not allowing random associations to derail our thought processes from their course. The canines, lesser apes, and humans (*Homosapiens sapiens sapiens*) do not represent successive stages on the same branch of the evolutionary tree. Nonetheless, they can be used as examples of different levels of development of the frontal lobes and of the correlation between frontal lobe development and the capacity for guiding behavior by internal representations, "the memories of the future."

When neurological illness affects the frontal lobes, the ability to stay on track becomes lost, and the patient is completely at the mercy of incidental environmental stimuli and tangential internal associations. It does not take much imagination to see how disruptive this disability can be. Easy distractability is a feature of many neurological and psychiatric disorders, and it is usually associated with frontal lobe dysfunction. As we will see later, attention deficit hyperactivity disorder (ADHD), with its extreme distractability, is usually linked to frontal lobe dysfunction.[24]

In psychiatry, susceptibility of thought processes to irrelevant associations has long been termed "tangentiality" and "loose association." These phenomena are among the most dramatic symptoms of schizophrenia. As we will see later, this is more than a coincidence. Schizophrenia today is regarded as a form of frontal lobe disease.

And then there is the everyday distractibility of the proverbial "absent-minded professor." Are we dealing with outright frontal lobe damage or with a variation of normal cognition? In the latter case, do the individual differences related to one's mental focus correspond to the individual differences in the "normal" function of the frontal lobes?

Rigidity of Mind

The ability to stay on track is an asset, but being "dead in the track" is not. One may very easily deteriorate into the other if the ability to maintain mental stability is not balanced by mental flexibility. No matter how focused we are on an activity or a thought, there comes a time when the situation calls for doing something else. Being able to change one's mindset is as important as staying mentally on track.

The capacity to switch with ease from one activity or idea to another is so natural and automatic that we take it for granted. In fact, it requires complex neural machinery, which also depends on the frontal lobes. Mental flexibility, the ability to see things in a new light, creativity, and originality all depend on the frontal lobes. When the frontal lobes are damaged, a certain "stiffness of the mind" sets in, and this too can be a very early manifestation of dementia.

We all occasionally encounter particularly inflexible people. We call them "rigid," and based on what we have already learned, their rigidity may be a "normal" individual variation of frontal lobe functions. More profound forms of mental rigidity produce obsessive-compulsive disorder (OCD), in which the dysfunction of the caudate nuclei closely linked to the frontal lobes has been implicated.[25] But outright frontal lobe damage produces extreme mental rigidity, which may completely paralyze the patient's cognition. This becomes strikingly clear when one watches Vladimir draw simple designs. In a regularly paced voice I dictate to Vladimir the names of the shapes to be drawn: "a cross, a circle, a square" and he draws them one by one following my instructions.

Stand back and think what this task entails. First, Vladimir has to decide whether the task requires *drawing* the shapes or *writing* their names. Based on our current knowledge of the brain, this task engages the language areas involved in the understanding of verb meaning, found immediately in front of Broca's area. Second, the meaning of the shape name has to be interpreted. This is accomplished in the left temporal lobe. Third, the image of the shape has to be accessed in long-term memory. Such images are probably stored in the temporal and parietal regions of the left hemisphere. Fourth, this image must be translated into a sequence of motor acts. This probably involves the premotor cortex. Fifth, each motor act must be executed. This is accomplished by the motor cortex. Sixth, the outcome of the action must be evaluated against the goal and the decision must be made whether the goal has been successfully accomplished. Finally, a smooth transition must be made to the next task and the cycle must be repeated. The last two tasks, evaluation and transition, are accomplished by the prefrontal cortex itself.[26] The outline of the cortical regions involved in the task are depicted in Figure 8.2.

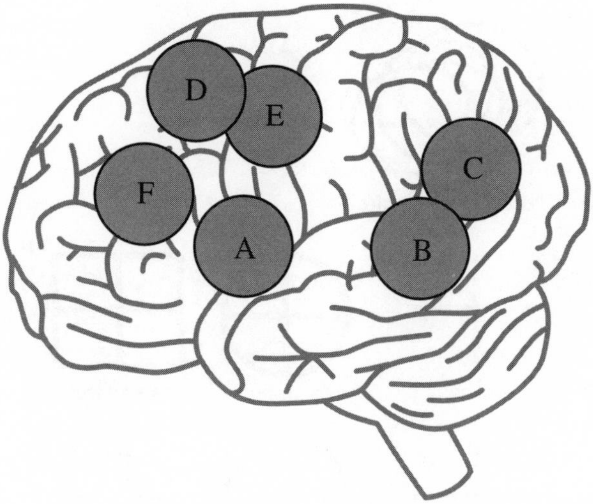

Figure 8.2. Cortical areas involved in drawing to dictation. (A) Decision is made whether the task requires *drawing* the shapes or *writing* their names. This task engages the area of the left frontal lobe found immediately in front of Broca's area. (B) The meaning of the shape name has to be interpreted. This is accomplished in the left temporal lobe. (C) The image of the appropriate shape has to be accessed in long-term memory. Such images are stored in the temporal and parietal regions of the left hemisphere. (D) The retrieved image must be translated into a sequence of motor acts. This involves the premotor cortex. (E) Each motor act must be executed. This is accomplished by the motor cortex. (F) The outcome of the action must be evaluated against the goal and the decision must be made whether the goal has been successfully accomplished. Finally, a smooth transition must be made to the next task and the cycle repeated. The last two tasks, evaluation and transition, are accomplished by the dorsolateral prefrontal cortex.

To pursue our orchestra analogy, even the seemingly simple task of drawing to dictation involves the concerted effort of several brain regions (the "players"), directed and supervised by the frontal lobes (the "conductor"). More complex behaviors require the coordinated action of far larger "ensembles"—also under the direction of the frontal lobes.

A closer look at a frontal patient's performance clarifies the relationship between the conductor and the orchestra. Complete transition from one task to another is impossible, and fragments of a previous task attach themselves to the new one, resulting in strange, hybrid designs. This phenomenon is called perseveration. Different kinds of *perseveration* are depicted in Figure 8.3.

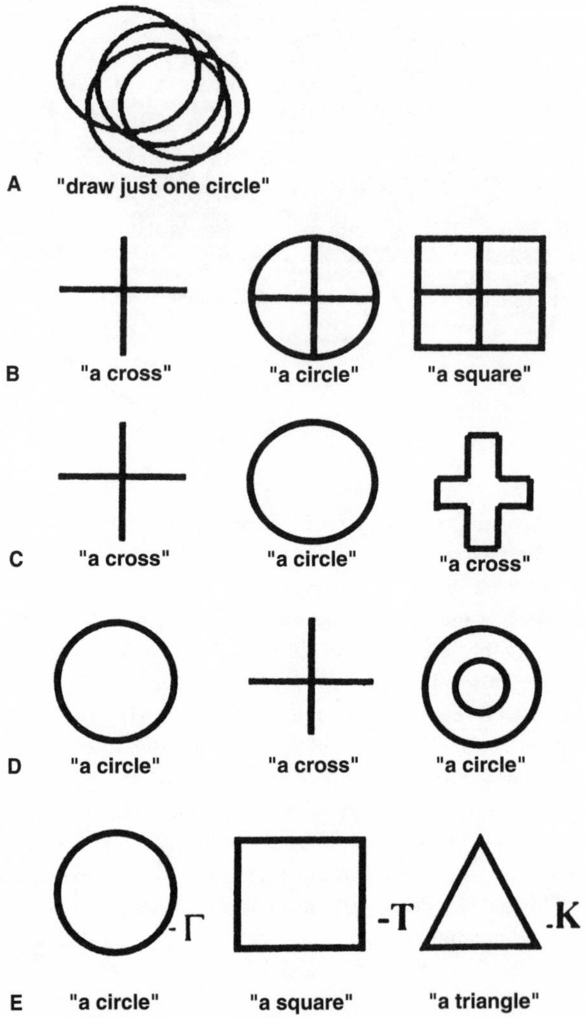

Figure 8.3. (A) Hyperkinetic perseveration reflects the failure of the prefrontal cortex to control motor output. (B) Perseveration of elements reflects the failure of the prefrontal cortex to control the output of premotor cortex. (C,D) Perseveration of features reflects the failure of the prefrontal cortex to control the output of the left posterior temporoparietal cortex. (E) Perseveration of activities reflects the breakdown of the prefrontal cortex itself. [For more detailed description see Goldberg and Tucker (1979). Reprinted by permission from Swets and Zeitlinger.]

In Vladimir's brain only the conductor, the frontal lobes, is damaged. All the players (the motor cortex, premotor cortex, and language areas in the left parietal and temporal lobes) are intact. Yet the performance of each player suffers as the result of frontal lobe damage. This is illustrated by the variety of forms that perseveration may take. Each of them reflects the failure of the frontal lobes to guide the behavior of a particular player. In other words, each type of perseveration in Figure 8.3 is caused by the breakdown of the executive control exerted by the frontal lobes over a distinct, far removed part of the cortex.

When asked to draw a circle (a loop requiring a single movement), a frontal patient keeps repeating the loop (Fig. 8.3A). This perseveration reflects the failure of the frontal lobes to guide the motor cortex.

When asked to draw a cross, a circle, and a square in sequence, the patient draws a cross and then, instead of "letting go" of it, attaches it to the circle and the square (Fig. 8.3B). Here a whole sequence of movements perseverates, rather than a single movement. This perseveration reflects the failure of the frontal lobes to guide the premotor cortex.

On a different occasion, the task is to draw a shape, a second shape, and then the first shape again. In Figure 8.3C, the first cross and the circle are drawn correctly, but the second cross acquires the property of the intervening circle—an area. In Figure 8.3D, the first circle is drawn correctly, but the second circle acquires the property of the intervening cross—"two-ness." These strange hybrids reflect the failure of the frontal lobes to select the mental representations of simple geometric forms stored in the temporal and parietal lobes and to complete the switch from one mental representation to the next one according to my instructions.

On a different occasion, the task was to draw a circle, a square, and a triangle, all of which the patient did well. He was then asked to write his name and his age. He did that too. Then he was again asked to draw a circle, a square, and a triangle. The result was a sequence of hybrid forms—half-shapes and half-letters (Fig. 8.3E). The juxtaposition of shapes and letters was not random. Attached to each shape was the terminal letter of its Russian name. In this task, the required sequence of activities was drawing–writing–drawing. With the frontal lobes failing to guide the process, this seemingly trivial transition could no longer be smoothly executed and the intervening writing impinged on the subsequent drawing, leading to hybrid performance. These hybrids reflect the failure of the frontal lobes to guide the interpretation of the verbal instruction given to the patient.[27]

Throughout the process, Vladimir was completely oblivious of his strange performance and unperturbed by its inconsistency. This is despite the fact that he remembered the task and could draw each of the shapes individually. Yet he was unable to compare the outcome of his labor to its goal.

The extreme inflexibility of mental operations evident in Vladimir's and other patients' performance is among the most devastating consequences of frontal lobe disease. In severe cases it is pervasive and it disrupts the work of virtually every other system in the brain. Vladimir's mental rigidity was extreme; yet in more subtle forms it permeates the mental processes of patients with even "mild" head trauma, early dementia, and other conditions. In those cases, the neurological basis of the symptoms is not always apparent. The subtle change in the patient's mental processes is often attributed to "personality" or "depression," when in fact subtle damage to the frontal lobes is present.

Vladimir's impairment exemplifies the effects of frontal lobe damage very well. He could not initiate activities. Having begun them, he could not terminate them. He could not form a plan; he could not follow a plan. His behavior was at the mercy of incidental distractions, both external and internal. He could not switch from one activity or thought to the next, and his mind became stuck. When, as the result of all these difficulties, his behavior became totally disintegrated, Vladimir lacked any awareness of his impairment.

At the same time, Vladimir's language was grammatically correct, as were his articulation and choice of words. He could read, write, and draw. He could engage is simple computations. His movements were unimpaired. His basic memory was intact. The musicians were spared. The conductor was gone.

Of course, Vladimir exhibited an extreme degree of mental rigidity. Nonetheless, his example captures the mechanism of a disorder which, even in much subtler forms, may deprive mental processes of their dynamism and agility. Loss of mental flexibility is among the very early, and difficult to recognize, manifestations of dementia.

A seemingly simple test turned out to be quite sensitive to subtle impairment of mental flexibility. The test, known as the Wisconsin Card Sorting Test,[28] requires the subject to sort cards with simple geometric forms into three categories according to a simple principle. The classification principle is not revealed in advance and the subject must establish it through trial and error. But when the principle is finally mastered it abruptly changes, unbeknownst to the subject. Once the subject catches up with the new principle, the principle is changed without forewarning again, and again, and again. The task requires planning, guidance by internal representation, mental flexibility, and working memory—in short all the aspects of frontal lobe function that we discussed before.

Mind Blindspot: Anosognosia

Our success in life critically depends on two abilities: the capacity for insight into our own mental world and that of other people. These abilities are closely interrelated and both are under frontal lobe control. Both abilities suffer following frontal lobe damage or poor development, and this leads to peculiar clinical syndromes. We already discussed the role of the frontal lobes in the ability to form insight into other people's minds, and how this ability suffers following damage to the frontal lobes. It is time now to consider the role of the frontal lobes in forming the insight into one's own cognitive world.

Again, Vladimir's case is very instructive. The most striking feature of Vladimir's condition was his complete unawareness of his disorder and of his drastically changed life circumstances. Vladimir suffered from *anosognosia*, a devastating condition which strips the patient of the capacity for insight into his own illness.[29] A patient with anosognosia may be severely impaired, yet he will have no inkling of it and will continue to claim that everything is fine. This is different from being "in denial," when it is assumed that the patient has the capacity to comprehend his own deficit but "chooses" to look the other way. Following frontal lobe damage the cognitive capacity for insight into one's own condition is genuinely lost.

Anosognosia may take many forms. For some reason, not fully understood, anosognosia is more common following damage to the right hemisphere than to the left hemisphere. Some scientists believe that this is because only language-mediated cognition is available for introspection, or because introspection itself is a language-based process. Therefore, according to this belief, any alteration of language-mediated cognitive processes due to brain damage would be available for introspection, and any alteration of nonverbal cognition due to brain damage would not be. This would limit the scope of introspection to left hemisphere–mediated mental processes.

I have always felt, however, that the connection of anosognosia with right but not left hemispheric lesions reflects a broader distinction between the functions of the two hemispheres.[30] The cognitive processes of the right hemisphere are less routinized, less dependent on stable codes, and involve more de novo computations. This is what makes their operational content less available to introspection, more "fuzzy" even in healthy individuals. Since the individual awareness of the right-hemispheric cognitive operations is "fuzzy" to begin with, their changes following brain damage are also less apparent.

Whatever the explanation, I find one patient, a successful international entrepreneur who suffered a massive right-hemispheric stroke, unforgettable. His performance on language tasks was perfectly intact, indicating the sparing of the left hemisphere. His performance on visuospatial tasks, requiring drawing or manipulation of visual forms devoid of meaning, was devastated, indicating severe damage to the right hemisphere. He was spatially disoriented to such a degree that he was completely unable to learn the layout of my modestly sized office and kept getting lost between the examination room, the reception area, and the bathroom. Yet he insisted that he had fully recovered, that nothing was the matter with him, and that he had to immediately fly to Cairo to finalize a business deal. There was no chance that he would have gotten anywhere near Cairo. He would have become hopelessly and completely lost the moment he got out of the taxicab at Kennedy International Airport. His wife and daughter understood this very well and, to their credit, arranged for his involuntary hospital admission despite his furious protestations.

But even this degree of anosognosia pales in comparison with the clinical picture common in severe frontal lobe damage. At least the traveling entrepreneur acknowledged that he had been ill. But Vladimir did not have a slightest inkling that his life had been catastrophically and irreversibly changed by the illness. No form of anosognosia is more complete and impermeable than the one caused by severe frontal lobe damage.[31]

The mechanisms of frontal lobe anosognosia are poorly understood. In a broad sense, they probably have to do with the impaired editorial function of the frontal lobes: comparing the outcome of one's operations with one's intentions. Or they may reflect an even deeper aspect of frontal lobe disease: the fundamental loss of intentionality inherent in it. An organism with no desires, no goals, no objectives will by definition experience no sense of failure. Awareness of the deficit is the basic prerequisite of any effort on the patient's behalf to improve his condition. A patient with anosognosia experiences no sense of loss or deficiency, and therefore no urge to strive to correct it. Since the patient's cooperation is critical to the success of any therapeutic effort, anosognosia turns the treatment process into an uphill battle, which makes the consequences of frontal lobe disease particularly devastating.

9

Social Maturity, Morality, Law, and the Frontal Lobes

Orbitofrontal "Pseudopsychopathic" Syndrome and the Loss of Self-Control

Among the myriad of anthropomorphic qualities lavished on the frontal lobes, they have been proclaimed the ultimate seat of morality. Does this mean that the underdevelopment of, or damage to, the frontal lobes will result in immorality? Probably not, but how about amorality?

Enter the orbitofrontal syndrome. The orbitofrontal syndrome is in many ways the opposite of the dorsolateral syndrome. The patients are emotionally disinhibited. Their affect is rarely neutral, constantly oscillating between euphoria and rage, with impulse control ranging from poor to nonexistent. Their ability to inhibit the urge for instant gratification is severely impaired. They do what they feel like doing when they feel like doing it, without any concern for social taboos or legal prohibitions. They have no foresight of the consequences of their actions.

A patient afflicted with the orbitofrontal syndrome (due to head injury, cerebrovascular illness, or dementia) will engage in shoplifting, sexually aggressive behavior, reckless driving, or other actions commonly perceived as antisocial. These patients are known to be selfish, boastful, puerile, profane, and sexually explicit. Their humor is off-color and their jocularity, known as *Witzelsucht,* resembles that of a drunken adolescent.[1] If the dorsolateral patients are in a sense devoid of personality, then orbitofrontal patients are conspicuous for their "immature" personality. Not surprisingly, European neurological science around 1900 dubbed the orbitofrontal syndrome the "pseudopsychopathic" syndrome. But in this case the untoward traits are caused by the damage to the orbitofrontal regions of the brain and are not under the patient's control.

The unkind term "pseudopsychopathic" is no longer in use. Although some patients with the orbitofrontal syndrome engage in criminally antisocial behaviors, most such patients come across as lacking in inhibitions, "loose" but harmless. Very often their disinhibition borders on the comical. An elderly patient walked into my office many years ago and said with a broad grin by way of greeting: "Doctor, you are a very hairy man!" Aside from this being untrue (I wish!), this is obviously no way to greet a stranger, who also happens to be your new doctor. My immediate diagnostic hunch was subsequently confirmed. The good man suffered from an early stage of dementia affecting particularly the frontal lobes.

In another case, an elderly wealthy country gentleman was brought by his wife to see me after he had bought 100 horses "on an impulse." He, too, was diagnosed with dementia, a relatively advanced one. When I asked the wife why she had not brought him to the doctor sooner, she conceded that he had been acting "silly" for the last few years, but she thought he was merely "sloshed" on his martinis. Both cases encapsulate the more benign form of "orbitofrontal disinhibition" (and the difficulty that lay people, even family members, have in recognizing it as a clinical disorder).

Society holds an individual responsible for certain actions but not for others. The scope of our responsibilities is defined by the scope of our volitional control. Vomiting in public by a drunk will be punished, but vomiting following a heat stroke will be excused. A traffic accident caused by speeding will be punished, but an accident caused by a driver's heart attack will be excused. Profanities spouted publicly in anger will be punished, but the same profanities uttered involuntarily by a coprolalic Tourette's patient might be excused. Bodily harm inflicted in assault will be punished, but bodily harm inflicted by a seizure patient who fell on a child will be excused.

Society draws a legal and moral distinction between the consequences of actions presumed to be under the individual's volitional control and those presumed to be outside such control. Drunkenness, speeding, rudeness, and aggression are usually presumed to be under volitional control, therefore avoidable and punishable. On the other hand, it is recognized that the effects of seizures, tics, fainting spells, and heart attacks cannot be controlled by the patient at the time of their happening, and therefore will not be punishable by law.

Volitional control implies more than conscious awareness. It implies the ability to anticipate the consequences of one's action, the ability to decide whether the action should be taken, and the ability to choose between action and inaction. A Tourette's patient and a hapless heatstroke-stricken vacationer may be fully aware of what is happening to them, but they cannot control it.

It appears that, at a cognitive level, the capacity for volitional behavior depends on the functional integrity of the frontal lobes. The capacity for restraint particularly depends on the orbitofrontal cortex.

Social Maturity and the Frontal Lobes

We recognize that the capacity for volitional control over one's actions is not innate, but that it emerges gradually through development. A temper tantrum thrown by an adult will trigger a very different reaction from a temper tantrum thrown by a child. The capacity for the volitional control over one's actions is an important, perhaps central, ingredient of social maturity.

Allan Schore, a psychiatrist from southern California, has proposed a provocative hypothesis.[2] He believes that early mother–infant interaction is important for the normal development of the orbitofrontal cortex during the first months of life. By contrast, early-life stressful experiences may permanently damage the orbitofrontal cortex, predisposing the individual to later-life psychiatric diseases.

If true, this is a mind-boggling proposition, since it implies that early social interactions help shape the brain. Scientists have known for years that early sensory stimulation promotes the development of visual cortex in the occipital lobes, and early life sensory deprivation retards its development. Is it possible that social stimulation is to the development of the frontal cortex what visual stimulation is to the development of the occipital cortex? A rigorous answer to this question may be hard to obtain in humans, but it lends itself to a pretty straightforward animal model. Aside from the role of early social interaction, I would like to see another question addressed: Is there a relationship between environmental orderliness (as opposed to chaotic environment) and the maturation of the frontal lobes? Given the role of the frontal lobes in the temporal organization of cognition, an early exposure to temporally ordered environments may prove to be crucial for this role to develop.

An even more audacious question may be asked: Is it possible that moral development involves the frontal cortex, just as visual development involves occipital cortex and language development involves temporal cortex? A moral code can be thought of as the taxonomy of sanctioned actions and behaviors. The prefrontal cortex is the association cortex of the frontal lobes, the "action lobes." Recall that the posterior association cortex encodes generic information about the outside world. It contains the taxonomy of the various things known to exist and helps recognize a particular exemplar as a member of a known category. Could it then be that, by analogy, the prefrontal cortex contains the taxonomy of all the *sanctioned, moral actions and behaviors*? And could it be that, just as damage or maldevelopment of the posterior association cortex produces *object agnosias*, so does damage or maldevelopment of the prefrontal cortex produce, in some sense, *moral agnosia*?

These far-reaching possibilities await further exploration, but a report by Antonio Damasio lends them some support. Damasio studied two young adults, a man and a woman, who suffered damage to the frontal lobes very early in life. Both engaged in antisocial behaviors: lying, petty thievery, truancy. Damasio claims that not only did these patients fail to act according to the proper, socially sanctioned moral precepts, but they even failed to recognize their actions as morally wrong.[3]

The orbitofrontal cortex is not the only part of the frontal lobes linked to socially mature behavior. The anterior cingulate cortex occupies a midfrontal position and is closely linked to the prefrontal cortex. Together with the prefrontal neocortex and the basal ganglia, the anterior cingulate cortex is part of what I like to call the "metropolitan frontal lobes." The anterior cingulate cortex has been traditionally linked to emotion. According to Michael Posner, the doyen of North American cognitive psychology, it also plays a role in social development by regulating distress.[4]

The ability to inhibit distress is fundamental to social interactions. The goals and needs of different members of a social group are never in perfect agreement, and the capacity for compromise is a critical mechanism of social harmony and equilibrium. This capacity depends on our ability to harness distress, the negative emotion arising from an inability to find immediate gratification. Negative emotions involve the amygdala, located deep within the temporal lobe. According to Posner, the anterior cingulate cortex reins in the amygdala, and by exerting this control tempers the expression of distress. A society of individuals with the active amygdala unrestrained by the anterior cingulate cortex would constantly be at each other's throats. According to this view, the anterior cingulate cortex makes civilized discourse and conflict resolution possible.

Biological Maturation and Social Maturity: A Historical Puzzle

The implicit definition of social maturity changes throughout the history of society, and so does the time of "coming of age." In various cultures the time when a boy becomes a man has been codified through rituals, and the change of this time in history is quite revealing.

In the Jewish tradition the age of 13 is celebrated by the *bar mitzvah.* In modern times, it is a joyous ritual full of symbolism. However, when the celebration is over, the boy remains a boy. The ritual of bar mitzvah probably reflects the reality of three millennia ago, when the age of 13 was the age of transition from boyhood to manhood with all its profound connotations.

Initiation rites symbolizing the passage into adulthood are also found in other cultures. On the Indonesian island of Bali, I observed the ceremony of *mepanes* (tooth filing). Mepanes is performed in late adolescence, around the age of 16, and is the prerequisite for entering any adult institution, such as marriage. Surrounded with colorful ritual heightened by the sound of ceremonial gamelans, the young man's or woman's teeth are filed by a *sangging* (a junior Hindu priest). The symbolism of the ritual is revealing.

Ida Bagus Madhe Adnyana, a young Brahmin who had his own teeth ritually filed a few years earlier, explained the meaning of the ceremony as follows. By acquiring flat and even teeth the teenager is set apart from animals, whose teeth are sharp and uneven. Flattening the teeth symbolizes joining the world of civilization. Six front upper teeth are filed, corresponding to six vices: *kama* (lust), *krodha* (anger), *lobha* (greed), *moha* (drunkenness), *mada* (arrogance), and *matsuya* (jealousy). Flattening the teeth symbolizes tempering these impulses and bringing them under the control of reason. We already know that many of these socially undesirable traits are tempered by the frontal lobes and become unmanageable with orbitofrontal injury.

As society became more complex and increasingly governed by brain rather than brawn, and as the life span increased, the age of maturity was pushed up. In modern Western societies the age of 18 (or thereabout) has been codified in the law as the age of social maturity. This is the age when a person can vote and is held responsible for his or her actions as an adult.

The age of 18 is also the age when the maturation of the frontal lobes is relatively complete. Various estimates can be used to measure the course of maturation of various brain structures. Among the most commonly used such measures is pathway myelinization.[5] Long pathways connecting different parts of the brain are covered with white fatty tissue called myelin.

Myelin insulates the pathway and speeds the neural signal transmission along the pathway. The presence of myelin makes communication between different parts of the brain faster and more reliable. Obviously, long-distance communication is particularly important for the frontal lobes, the CEO of the brain, since their role is to coordinate the activities of its many parts. The frontal lobes cannot fully assume their leadership role until the pathways connecting the frontal lobes with the far-flung structures of the brain are fully myelinated.

The agreement between the age of relatively complete maturation of the frontal lobes and the age of social maturity is probably more than coincidental. Without the explicit benefit of neuroscience, but through cumulative everyday common sense, society recognizes that an individual assumes adequate control over his or her impulses, drives, and desires only by a certain age. Until that age, an individual cannot be held fully responsible for his actions in either a legal or a moral sense. This ability appears to depend critically on the maturity and functional integrity of the frontal lobes.

The relationship between the age of social maturity and the maturation of the frontal lobes through history raises interesting questions. In ancient and medieval societies social adulthood was achieved at a much earlier age than it is today. Kingdoms were often ruled, and armies routinely led into battle, by teenagers. Pharaoh Ramses the Great of Egypt, the biblical King David, and Alexander the Great of Macedon all embarked on their major military campaigns while in their early twenties. In fact, Alexander was barely 20 when he crossed the Bosphorus, invaded Persia, and by this act began the fusion of East and West. He was dead at 32, having created one of the greatest empires on earth, from modern-day Libya to India. Peter the Great of Russia set about tearing down and transforming his country while in his late teens. By all available accounts, none of these historical figures was a puppet in somebody else's, more "mature" hands. Each was a decisive, visionary leader of his people at a very young age, and each of them left an indelible trace on civilization. Yet in most developed countries today people their age are prevented from occupying high offices by law, on the assumption of their "immaturity." By law, a president of the United States must be at least 35, which would have disqualified many great historical political figures from occupying the leadership position in our society.

Does this mean that some of the most important decisions in history were made by biologically immature brains? To take it a step further, could it be that much of human history is the neurological equivalent of a juvenile mob scene, and that the most fateful conflicts in ancient and medieval history are best modeled on William Golding's *Lord of the Flies*?[6] The role of elders as arbitrators, moderators, and generally "wise men" was paramount in ancient societies. Is it because the elders were the bearers of neurological, and not just social, maturity?

Or is it possible that the biological rate of frontal lobe maturation is at least partly controlled by environmental (and in the human case cultural) factors, such as an early pressure to assume "adult" roles and engage in complex decision making (a hypothesis proposed by my student John Solerno)? The frontal lobe nature–nurture question is interesting both for theoretical and practical reasons in this age of rapid social change. Obviously, we do not have brain-imaging data from the times of antiquity. Nor does the idea of imaging the brains of the youthful tribal chiefs in the few remaining primitive societies in the Amazon jungle or Papua New Guinea highlands seem particularly practical. But nonhuman primate experimentation may help answer the question.

Frontal Lobe Damage and Criminal Behavior

We all behave in impulsive and irresponsible ways at times, but most of us have the ability to stay clear of outright criminality. By contrast, behavior devoid of social inhibitions for neurological reasons is much more likely to cross the line. Extreme violations of human norms of behavior intuitively strike us as abnormal; that they are "abnormal' by definition is a truism. It is not by coincidence that we use the word "sick" to describe such behaviors. Instinctively, we refuse to accept them as part of "normal" behavior and try to understand them in "clinical" terms. One reads speculations about Lenin's and Idi Amin's tertiary syphilis, Stalin's paranoia, Hitler's von Economo's encephalitis, and so on. But by inflating the concept of criminal insanity, we devalue fundamental legal and ethical concepts. One must tread very carefully in drawing the line between criminality and mental illness, between morality and biology.

The relationship between frontal lobe damage and criminality is particularly intriguing and complex. We already know that damage to the frontal lobes causes the impairment of insight, impulse control, and foresight, which often leads to socially unacceptable behavior. This is particularly true when the damage affects the orbital surface of the frontal lobes. Patients afflicted with this "pseudopsychopathic" syndrome are notorious for their urge for instant gratification, they are unrestrained by social mores or fear of punishment. It would be logical to suspect that some of these patients are particularly prone to criminal behavior. But is there any evidence? More important, is there any evidence that some of the individuals indicted, convicted, or sentenced for criminal behavior are, in fact, unrecognized cases of frontal lobe damage?

Several marginal groups in society exhibit the peculiar trait of relinquishing their executive functions to external institutions, where their options are maximally constrained and the decision-making power over them is exercised by someone else. Some chronic psychiatric patients feel uncomfortable outside mental institutions and seek readmission; some criminals feel uncomfortable in the outside world and seek ways for being reincarcerated. This could be construed as a peculiar form of self-medication, as an attempt to compensate for an executive deficit rendering them incapable of making their own decisions.

It has been suggested, based on several published studies, that the prevalence of head injury is much higher among criminals than in the general population, and in violent criminals than in nonviolent criminals.[7] For reasons of brain and skull anatomy, closed head injury is particularly likely to affect the frontal lobes directly, especially the orbitofrontal cortex. But later in this book I will argue that direct damage to the frontal lobes is not even necessary to produce significant frontal lobe dysfunction. Damage to the upper brain stem is likely to produce a similar effect by interrupting the critical projections into the frontal lobes. Damage to the upper brain stem is extremely common in closed head injury, even in seemingly "mild" cases, and it is likely to produce frontal lobe dysfunction even in the absence of direct damage to the frontal lobes. Many years ago I described this condition under the name of the "reticulofrontal disconnection syndrome."[8]

Contemporary research bears out the designation of certain frontal lobe syndromes as "pseudopsychopathic." Adrian Raine and his colleagues studied the brains of convicted murderers with positron emission tomography (PET) scan and found abnormalities in the prefrontal cortex.[9] Raine and colleagues also studied the brains of men with antisocial personality disorder and found an 11% reduction in the gray matter of their frontal lobes.[10] The cause of this reduction is uncertain, but Raine believes that this reduction is at least in part congenital, as opposed to being caused by environmental factors such as abuse or bad parenting.

If this assertion is true, then it appears that people with certain congenital forms of brain dysfunction may be particularly predisposed to antisocial behavior. On the face of it, this assertion is not implausible. We have long recognized the existence of congenital predisposition to brain dysfunction due to aberrant patterns of neural cell migration and other causes. But it is only logical to assume that such "genotypic" predisposition can be quite broad and devoid of neuroanatomical specificity and that its individual "phenotypic" expressions are highly variable and may affect different parts of the brain in different individuals. Just as in certain cases this predisposition may affect the temporal lobe leading to language-based learning disability, so in other cases it may affect the prefrontal cortex producing a "social learning disability" of sorts.

The link between frontal lobe dysfunction and asocial behavior raises an important legal issue. Suppose a criminal is found to have structural evidence of frontal lobe damage on magnetic resonance imaging (MRI) or computerized axial tomography (CAT) scan; or suppose physiological evidence of frontal lobe dysfunction is found on PET, single photon emission computerized tomography (SPECT), or electroencephalography (EEG). These are all commonly used and widely available diagnostic neuroimaging devices. Or suppose that a criminal is found to perform particularly poorly on the neuropsychological tests sensitive to the function of the frontal lobes.

Suppose, further, that the nature of the crime suggests spur-of-the-moment impulsivity and lack of premeditation. (Obviously, premeditation and intricate planning would argue strongly against severe frontal lobe dysfunction.) In a legal sense, a "frontal" patient may be competent to stand trial, since he can understand the court proceedings. Rhetorically, he may also know right from wrong, and will correctly answer the questions about which actions are socially acceptable and which are not. In all likelihood, the patient would have had this knowledge available to him in a token form even at the time of the crime. Therefore, the insanity defense will not be conventionally applicable. Yet the frontal damage would interfere with his ability to parlay this knowledge into a socially acceptable course of action. Although the difference between right and wrong is known, the knowledge cannot be translated into effective inhibitions.

The discrepancy between rhetorical knowledge and the ability to utilize this knowledge for guiding behavior is conspicuous in frontal lobe patients. This can be demonstrated very dramatically with a simple bedside test introduced by Alexandr Luria.[11] A patient is seated in front of the examiner and asked to do the opposite of what the examiner does: "When I raise my finger, you raise your fist. When I raise my fist, you raise your finger." This task is particularly difficult for frontal lobe patients. Instead of doing "the opposite," they tend to lapse into direct imitation. To help the patient with the task, one may encourage him to say aloud what needs to be done. At this point the disparity between rhetorical knowledge and the ability to guide behavior with this knowledge becomes strikingly obvious. The patient will say the right thing but make the wrong move at the same time. With my colleagues and former students Bob Bilder, Judy Jaeger, and Ken Podell, I developed the Executive Control Battery, a collection of tests to elicit precisely such phenomena.[12]

An orbitofrontal patient may know right from wrong yet be unable to use this knowledge to regulate his behavior. Likewise, a mesiofrontal patient with damage to the anterior cingulate cortex will know the rules of civilized behavior but will be unable to *follow them.* The potential legal ramifications of this condition are vast, and the recognition of this possibility represents a legal new frontier.

What is the likelihood of an asocial individual suffering from some form of orbitofrontal or mesiofrontal dysfunction? Under what conditions should this possibility be directly ascertained through neuropsychological and neuroimaging means? What is the legal significance of such evidence? When does it override criminal responsibility? Two legal decisions rest on cognitive evidence: (1) Is the defendant competent to stand trial, and (2) Is the defendant sufficiently sane to be held criminally responsible for his or her actions? Based on the standard criteria used in courts in such decisions, a frontal lobe patient may be pronounced both legally competent and legally sane. But whether these legal constructs adequately cover the peculiar potential for asocial behavior related to frontal lobe damage is arguable. The third relevant legal concept is "diminished capacity." This broad concept may be applicable by virtue of its vagueness, but for the same reason it eludes clear-cut criteria to guide legal decision making.

At the time of this writing, a bizarre criminal case was unfolding in New York. An obstetrician had carved his initials into a woman's belly after performing a caesarean section. According to the press reports, when challenged, the doctor said nonchalantly that he felt that his surgery had been such a masterpiece that he had to sign it; then he took off on vacation to Paris. As soon as I read about the incident in the *New York Times*, I said to myself that it was too bizarre, too "sick" to be "merely" criminal. And true enough, as a defense, the doctor's attorneys claimed that he suffered from frontal lobe damage due to Pick's disease.

Curiously, the mutilated woman—also a doctor—opposed the obstetrician's criminal prosecution, evidently recognizing that his behavior had been more tragic than criminal. The doctor would have faced up to 25 years in prison had he been convicted of the most serious charge brought up by the prosecution, first-degree assault. Instead, he was sentenced to five years' probation and barred from applying for a medical license for five years. It is unlikely that he will ever attempt to practice medicine again.

A new legal construct of "inability to guide one's behavior despite the availability of requisite knowledge" may be needed to capture the peculiar relationship between frontal lobe dysfunction and the potential for criminal behavior. Studies of frontal lobe disorders bring into a single focus neuropsychology, ethics, and law. As the legal profession becomes more enlightened about the workings of the brain, the "frontal lobe defense" may emerge as a legal strategy on a par with the "insanity defense."

The exact limits of such a defense have yet to be tested and its legitimate boundaries established. It is almost inevitable that attempts will be made to stretch it beyond its legitimate boundaries. On the other hand, constructive multidisciplinary debate will be fostered. Is it possible that certain types of subtle frontal lobe dysfunction may render an individual amoral while sparing his capacity for planning and temporal organization (admittedly a far-fetched conjecture, but an interesting one)? In that case, is it a likely mechanism of sociopathy ("moral blindness")? Is it possible that sociopathic behavior may be caused by a neurodevelopmental disorder of the frontal lobes, just as dyslexia may be caused by a neurodevelopmental disorder of the temporal lobe? Are we trivializing and debasing the notion of morality by setting on this path, or merely pointing to its "biological basis"? Are we further diluting the notion of personal responsibility? Or are we finally acknowledging that whereas moral and criminal codes are extracranial, moral and criminal cognition and behaviors are not? They are the products of our cerebral machinery, intact or abnormal, every bit as much as they are the products of our social institutions.

The Hapless Robber

Charlie was a happy-go-lucky guy and everybody's friend, bright and personable, who dropped out of school, got a job, and earned his grade school equivalency diploma. His parents, upright people from rural Pennsylvania, encouraged him to join the marines to keep him "on the straight and narrow." Charlie joined, served, was discharged, returned to Pennsylvania, and got a job as a salesman.

Then, at the age of 25, his very ordinary life was shattered in a single instant. One night, when Charlie and a friend were returning from a party, their open vehicle rammed into the metal support of a small bridge. Charlie's friend, the driver, was killed instantly and Charlie was found unconscious in a pool of blood on the side of the road.

Charlie did not regain consciousness until two and a half months later. Then he began several months of cognitive and physical therapy in a rehabilitation hospital. Several CAT scans conducted right after the accident showed signs of damage in the right temporal lobe and in the brain stem, general swelling (edema) of the brain, and blood in the lateral ventricles. There were also multiple skull fractures, including a basal skull fracture. A CAT scan repeated six years later showed substantial but incomplete recovery. It was probably damage to the upper brain stem, and the consequent reticulofrontal disconnection syndrome, that was largely responsible for all Charlie's troubles which followed. The presence of basal skull fracture also raised the possibility of direct damage to the orbitofrontal brain regions, even though it was not seen on CAT scans.

Released from the hospital, Charlie returned to his mother's home (his parents had been divorced for some time) and embarked on an idle, vacuous existence. He spent his days watching television, drinking beer, and taking drugs. Eventually, in a state of total exasperation, his mother threw him out. Charlie's father took him in, but not for long. One day Charlie brought home a woman with Tourette's syndrome and the two settled in his grandmother's bed. The woman's noisy tics gave the lovers away, and Charlie was told to leave again.

Charlie married the woman with Tourette's and embarked on a chaotic existence. At times he lived in the woman's house. At other times Charlie hit the road, wandering around the country, drunk and drugged much of the time, occasionally engaging in petty robberies. Charlie had recovered his physical faculties and, to a superficial observer, his mental faculties also. He was reasonably articulate and had no obvious stigma of a neurologically impaired patient. Despite his wild ways, he was generally a good-natured fellow. He had a short fuse, however, and got into arguments easily. Charlie occasionally found menial jobs, but he could never hold one for long and ended up on the road again.

Charlie was able to get by until one day he ran out of cash and decided to hold up a convenience store. In this pursuit, Charlie enlisted the help of a companion, also brain-damaged, whom he had met earlier at the rehabilitation hospital. Pointing a Bic lighter through his pants pocket in lieu of a gun, Charlie was able to get some $200 in cash. With the holdup in progress, his partner in crime was patiently waiting in the escape car in front of the store, the license plates fully exposed. Charlie was tracked down and arrested within two hours of the robbery, as he was settling down to enjoy the booze and the drugs acquired with the illgotten money.

Charlie's misadventure is an excellent example of "frontal lobe crime," precisely because of his utter ineptness. The most remarkable feature of the whole episode is a total lack of precision, foresight, or contingency planning. The crime was so pathetically bungled that it engendered more pity than outrage.

The court was unaware of Charlie's brain damage and he went to jail. Although the prison officers were also unaware of Charlie's neurological condition, he was perceived as "odd" and spent most of the time in the prison infirmary until he was let out on parole. This time his aging mother made the connection between Charlie's behavior and his old brain damage. Charlie was placed in a long-term rehabilitation center run by my former student Dr. Judith Carman. This is where I met him.

Trim and neatly dressed, Charlie did not carry the stigma of a neurological patient. He entered Dr. Carman's office with an athletic stride and a friendly smile, nothing in his demeanor betraying either the history of brain damage or the history of crime. Superficially articulate and gregarious, he offered no obvious hint at a cognitive deficit. He seemed to be self-conscious about his appearance, immediately challenging me to guess his age (he was 42 but looked younger), and asked me whether I liked his goatee.

Charlie knew that I was the program director's former professor, was writing a book, and wanted to include Charlie's story in it. He had been expecting our meeting for some time and was determined to put his best foot forward. He was quite excited about being in my book, and he was disappointed to find out that it would take me a while to finish it. He kept prodding me: "C'mon, get on with it, doc!" Charlie proceeded with a jolly delivery of his life's story, dwelling on its more delinquent details with particular relish, and sprinkling his narrative with casual profanities. This left the uncanny impression of a tipsy teenager in the body of a middle-aged man, the famous orbitofrontal *Witzelsucht.*

> "Do you like it here in this program?" I asked
> "No."
> "Why not?"
> " 'Cause I am horny, doc, and this witch [points at Dr. Carman with a grin suggesting that his choice of the word is a concession to my presence] isn't much help . . . Do you have any daughters for me, doc?" [slaps me on the knee, winks, and laughs genially] . . . "You don't mind my free thinking, do you?"

Charlie is known at the center for his roving eye and fancies the idea of marrying one of the center's female residents (he has been divorced from his tourettic wife for some time), because "once you fall off the horse you get right back on it." Charlie's sexual tension took a variety of forms. Once he somehow obtained lollypops in the shape of a penis and went around offering them to the center's female employees. Charlie recounted the episode fondly and with flourish, laughing at the memories of the scandalized women, and referring to the lollypops as "dick candy," not in the least inhibited by Dr. Carman's presence.

In the course of the conversation Charlie casually put his hand on Dr. Carman's behind. When asked to account for his behavior, Charlie's answer was that "it [his hand] just happened to be in motion." While this explanation would have sounded gratuitous coming from a neurologically intact individual, Charlie had unwittingly captured the essence of his condition. In Charlie the *it,* or shall we say the *id,* was no longer under an effective neural control by the frontal lobes.

Yet his upright preaccident background came through in incongruous ways. When one of the therapists suggested that he might consider doing what men have done since the beginning of time lacking female companionship, Charlie was first appalled by the idea, since it was contrary to his Christian upbringing. I am told that he has since adopted a more secular view of his options, and his life at the rehabilitation center has been more under control.

Much as Charlie would like to talk about sex, I changed the subject, asking "Do you feel that you have recovered from your accident?"

"Nobody recovers from an accident 100%, but let us say 99.9%," he said.

But then came a stunningly eloquent revelation, demonstrating more insight into his circumstances than Charlie's bravado would suggest:

"Head injury is like an eternal spring of youth. It stops you from growing up. It happened to me at 25 and I still feel 25 . . . A 42-year old would have more common sense . . ."

But Charlie seems to enjoy his "eternal spring of youth" and the insight proves to be shallow: "The car accident was a blessing . . ."

This surreal conversation coming to an end, Charlie gave me a tour of his room, with photographs of family members and two tanks with exotic fish. I kept thinking that he was a warm, genial person without a hint of malice or deceit, a teenager in a grown man's body, that despite his crude language there was a certain charm and innocence about him, and that I liked him. We shook hands and he slapped me on the back, reminding me to send him a copy of the book.

At the time of this writing, Charlie continues to live at the rehabilitation center and work in the community. Jobs are found for him through a placement program run at the center. Most of the time Charlie is a conscientious worker and does a good job fixing and cleaning things. He tends to get into trouble with his employers, however, because of his short fuse and loose tongue. His uninhibited behavior got him fired from his previous job and he is now a janitor in a department store. Now and then Charlie transgresses, like when he stole the center's car and went for a ride (he does not have a valid driver license).

Most of the time Charlie is an amiable fellow and has no intention of hurting anyone. He is generally funny and gregarious. But true to his orbitofrontal syndrome, Charlie has a volatile temper, which tends to bounce precipitously from one extreme to the other. If someone is in his way, he is likely to turn around and punch that person out without warning or deliberation. And since Charlie has physically recovered from his injury and now lifts weights for recreation, he is capable of doing real damage. It does not take much provocation to get Charlie going. When another center resident appropriated his ice cream by mistake, Charlie's fists began to flash in a scary fit of rage, and it took four people to subdue him.

Under the circumstances, Charlie's recovery was quite remarkable. He is athletic and articulate, showing no obvious memory impairment. Today, most people would think of Charlie as "odd," "immature," "loose cannon," "obnoxious," or "vulgar." But very few people would realize that Charlie is brain-damaged. I suspect that many psychologists and physicians would miss that also. The neuropsychological evaluations administered repeatedly several years after the accident suggested average intelligence (Wechsler Adult Intelligence Scale–Revised IQ values within the 90s) and low average memory (Wechsler Memory Scale–Revised values within the 80s).[13] Charlie's performance on language tests was also within a normal range. All the test results were probably lower than they would have been without the accident, but nothing in them betrayed the extent of Charlie's injuries. Yet Charlie's core was gone and so was his mooring. Charlie's case captures the essence of the frontal lobe syndrome: specific skills spared but inner guide gone.

Frontal Lobe Damage and the Public Blindspot

Charlie's story is instructive in more ways than one. For years Charlie moved in and out of menial jobs, lived intermittently with various people, and nobody suspected that Charlie's oddities had a neurological cause. This is notwithstanding the fact that many people around him knew about Charlie's accident.

This raises the broad issue of general public awareness of cognitive impairment. Although rhetorically the educated public understands today that cognition is a function of the brain, this abstraction often fails to inform specific, real-life situations. As a result, Cartesian dualism is alive and well when it comes to everyday encounters with brain-damaged people. This naive dualism is evident even at the level of health care policymaking and health coverage, when physical health is treated seriously while "mental" health is given short shrift.

Everyday public attitudes betray a sharp division between "physical" and "nonphysical" symptoms and between "physical" and "nonphysical" bodily organs. Problems with vision or hearing, limp, weakness on one side of the body will be unfailingly perceived as physical and will engender sympathy and readiness to help. The bodily nature of these symptoms will be immediately grasped, but curiously, most lay people will be very slow attributing them to the brain.

By contrast, patients with higher-order cognitive impairments are often denied the sympathy accorded people with physical infirmities and are treated instead in moralistic, almost puritanical terms.

Forget the hapless criminal Charlie. Consider the common situation of a demented elderly individual whose whole life has been an example of civic responsibility and moral rectitude. Now she is old and very forgetful. Having diagnosed early dementia, I am trying to explain the implications of my findings to the eager family members. I tell them that their mother suffers from amnesia, that her forgetfulness is caused by brain atrophy, that she cannot help it, that it is likely to get worse, and that they have to be patient with their loved one. The family members listen intently. They nod. They seem to understand—and then comes an irate comment: "But how come I give her breakfast in the morning and she comes back asking for her breakfast again!" When I encounter this lack of understanding, I feel like tipping my hat (not that I wear one) to my friend Oliver Sacks, who has done more than anyone else to enlighten the general public about the effects of neurological injury on cognition. I urge people to read *The Man Who Mistook His Wife for a Hat.*[14]

But if the neurological nature of impaired memory, perception, or language usually can be grasped by the general public, the executive deficit caused by frontal lobe injury almost never is grasped. Point to the patient's impulsivity, volatility, indifference, lack of initiative, and the common response will be "This is not his brain, this is his personality!" This is total retreat three and a half centuries back to Cartesian dualism, as if "personality" were an utterly extracranial phenomenon. And the notion of "personality," of course, is something that, on a par with apple pie and spring water, carries moralistic, righteous connotations. If you were born into an honest family and went to a good school, then how dare you not have an upright personality!

It is my hope that this book will help put "personality" and related expressions of the mind where they belong, inside the brain, so to speak, in the eyes of the general public. By helping accomplish this, the book will help correct the unintended public insensitivity, and sometimes outright cruelty, toward the most devastating of all forms of brain damage, the damage to the frontal lobes.

10

Fateful Disconnections

The Fallen Horseman: A Case Study

When my neurosurgeon friend Jim Hughes called late at night, as was his habit, I had no notion that the consequences of this call would profoundly affect my career. Jim wanted me to consult on his patient, a man in his late thirties recovering from a head injury. It sounded like a pretty routine clinical case and I agreed to see the patient.

Kevin (a fictional name) was a fabulously successful entrepreneur and entertainment executive, a happy husband and father of three. An all-round athlete, he was an accomplished equestrian, but that day he was riding an unfamiliar horse in New York's Central Park and was thrown on hard basalt rock, hitting his head against a tree in the process. He was rushed to the nearest hospital, where Dr. Hughes performed emergency surgery. Kevin had been comatose for two days and was slowly recovering.

I first saw Kevin briefly approximately two months after his accident. He was disoriented, confused, and overwhelmed by his surroundings. His general demeanor was panic-stricken, and if there ever was an embodiment of the expression "shell-shocked," Kevin was that embodiment. He was severely aphasic and responded to every question addressed to him by saying "Thank you . . . thank you . . . thank you." That was his only utterance. There was something extremely childlike and pleading in his demeanor and his "thank you"—he was a man who had lost his core, defenseless like a child. I was struck by the thought that in some metaphoric sense he was in a fetal position, even though he was not. He wandered aimlessly on the unit walking through any open door—just because the door was there. He was very thin, almost emaciated, the hair on his head barely beginning to grow back after neurosurgery. Nothing in this fragile visage was evocative of the supremely confident, buoyant, and physically imposing persona that the old Kevin was supposed to have been.

Kevin was discharged from the hospital, and three months later I was asked to see him again. He was a different person, his wavy hair regrown into a rich mane, his weight regained, with a broad smile on his face and gregarious manners returned. His language was fluent and his mood relaxed. Dressed in one of his expensive suits, his hair blown dry, Kevin appeared the epitome of a palpably successful dweller of New York's Upper East Side. Superficially, his demeanor of a man in control of his environment had returned, and one could imagine the old Kevin—a self-confident, charismatic, and slightly glib, upper-crust New Yorker.

In reality, Kevin was far from recovered. He still had significant memory impairment, which affected both his ability to learn new information (anterograde amnesia) and his ability to recall information learned well before his accident (retrograde amnesia). His language, while generally fluent and even articulate, revealed slight word-finding difficulties, maybe not likely to be noticed by the uninitiated, but certainly apparent to me.

As I continued to observe Kevin, I was particularly struck by the severity of his "frontal lobe syndrome." Kevin was perseverative; that is, his behavior invariably fell into repetitive stereotypes. Every evening, he would arrange his clothes for the following day and the clothes were always the same. As winter passed and spring began, and well into the summer, Kevin continued to prepare his sheepskin jacket to wear the following day and could be found walking around the Upper East Side of Manhattan clad in his sheepskin on a sweltering July day. It took a lot of persuasion to get him to wear anything else. Despite his superficial flair, any conversation with Kevin rapidly deteriorated into a rather vacuous activity such as simple card games. He had a small repertoire of rehearsed stock topics, and the conversation would predictably and quickly drift toward one of them, say, discussion of some of his friends. Having run through his repertoire of half-a-dozen topics, Kevin would start from the beginning, repeating everything almost verbatim again and again.

Kevin was not only perseverative, but he was also field-dependent. Accompanied by a family member or an aide, Kevin occasionally ventured into a neighborhood restaurant for lunch. In the restaurant he tended to order every item on the menu, 10 or 20 items in all. He did so not because he was that hungry, but because the items were there. He spent most of his time, though, languishing in his apartment, occasionally asking people to play simple card games and backgammon with him. His behavior during the games was childlike. He would clap his hands with joy after winning and throw temper tantrums after losing. He was not above cheating.

Kevin's affect was constantly oscillating between euphoria and superficial rage. These mood swings were abrupt, extreme, and could be precipitated by the most trivial events—like a waitress in a restaurant asking him if he wanted more coffee.

His personality took on childlike characteristics in virtually every respect. He related to his wife like a 12-year old and competed with his children for her attention. In many ways he interacted with his children as an equal. Like a little child, he demanded instant gratification, although his needs were not those of a child. On several occasions he approached his female acquaintances with rather explicit propositions, an odd combination of the old charming Kevin and the socially inappropriate frontal patient.

Kevin had no insight into his condition. When questioned about the effects of the accident, he would mention his physical injuries but maintained that his mind was sound. He was convinced that he was ready to go back to work. When asked why he had not done so, he would say that he did not feel like it, or that he had been busy doing other things. Eventually Kevin was encouraged to spend a few hours a day in his old office, engaged in various cognitive exercises designed to help his recovery. He enjoyed going to the office and chatting with his old colleagues. His sense was that he was "back to work"—despite the fact that the way he spent his time in the office bore little similarity with his activities before the accident.

Kevin's mind was astoundingly concrete. When I once said that it was time to repeat the CAT (computerized axial tomography) scan, this was met with genuine puzzlement. Why the CAT scan, Kevin marveled, if after all he had been hurt by a horse, not a cat? On another occasion, somebody used the metaphor "increasingly interconnected isles of communications" to refer to the growing role of communications in North America. This threw Kevin into a fit of rage, since the United States "has never consisted of a bunch of islands."

The more time I spent with Kevin, the more convinced I became that his cognition was a textbook case of the "frontal lobe syndrome." The puzzling thing was that not a single one of the several CAT scans administered to Kevin could detect a frontal lobe lesion. This is not to say that Kevin's brain was normal; far from it. Kevin suffered severe and multiple brain damage.

The damage affected the temporoparietal regions in both hemispheres. The ventricles (spaces within the brain containing cerebrospinal fluid) were enlarged. There was also a shunt surgically placed in his brain to help the drainage of cerebrospinal fluid. But the frontal lobes were clear—an amazing finding in a patient with such strong clinical evidence of frontal lobe dysfunction.

The discrepancy between the clinical picture of Kevin's behavior and his CAT scans presented an intellectual challenge and Kevin became another important patient on my career path who influenced, and even shaped, its direction. With the help of my research assistants Bob Bilder and Carl Sirio (now a prominent neuropsychologist and a prominent physician, respectively), I embarked on a detective mission of sorts, trying to unravel the mystery of Kevin's condition. Since no such condition had ever been described before, we were on our own.

If the frontal lobes themselves were structurally intact, I reasoned, is it possible that the problem lay with the pathways connecting them to some other structures? Could it be a frontal disconnection syndrome? The concept of a "disconnection syndrome" was introduced by Norman Geschwind,[1] one of the preeminent American behavioral neurologists, whose numerous students continue to shape the field. The idea was that a severe cognitive deficit could be caused not by the damage to a brain structure per se, but by the damage to long connecting nerve fibers between two brain structures, interrupting the information flow between them. But the classic disconnection syndromes were "horizontal," affecting the connections between two or more cortical regions. I had the inkling that in Kevin's case we encountered a "vertical" disconnection syndrome. Could it be that Kevin's condition was caused by damage to the massive pathways projecting from the brain stem into the frontal lobes?

The brain stem contains the nuclei thought to be responsible for the arousal and activation of the rest of the brain. Collectively some of these nuclei are called the "reticular formation," a bit of a misnomer and a conceptual anachronism, since the term implies a diffuse undifferentiated action. Today we know that the reticular formation consists of distinct components, each with its own biochemical properties.

The complex relationship that exists between the frontal lobes and the brain stem reticular nuclei is best described as a loop. On the one hand, the arousal of the frontal lobes depends on the ascending pathways from the brain stem. These pathways are complex, but one component—the mesocortical dopamine system—is thought to be particularly important for the proper function of the frontal lobes. It originates in the ventral tegmental area (VTA) of the brain stem and projects into the frontal lobes. If the frontal lobes are the decision-making center of the brain, then the ventral tegmental area is its energy source, the battery, and the ascending mesocortical dopamine pathway is the connecting cable.

On the other hand, there are pathways projecting from the frontal lobes to the reticular nuclei of the ventral brain stem. Through these pathways the frontal lobes exert their control over the diverse brain structures by modulating their arousal level. If the frontal lobes are the decision-making device, then the reticular formation is an amplifier helping communicate these decisions to the rest of the brain in a loud and clear voice. The descending pathways are the cables through which the instructions flow from the frontal lobes to the critical ventral brain stem nuclei.

I suspected that as a result of the accident a small lesion occurred in Kevin's brain somewhere along these pathways, probably in the ventral upper brain stem, where the critical pathways originate. Even a small lesion in that area could produce a devastating effect, and it could easily remain undetected by the relatively crude, first-generation CAT scans available to us at the time. On the strength of this hunch, we ordered a new CAT scan and asked the radiologists to examine the brain stem with the highest resolution possible. And there it was, a lesion sitting exactly in the ventral tegmental area and effectively destroying it (Fig. 10.1). I called this condition the "reticulofrontal disconnection syndrome."[2]

As I am writing this book 20 years after my encounter with Kevin, I think that on balance he did more for us, his doctors, than

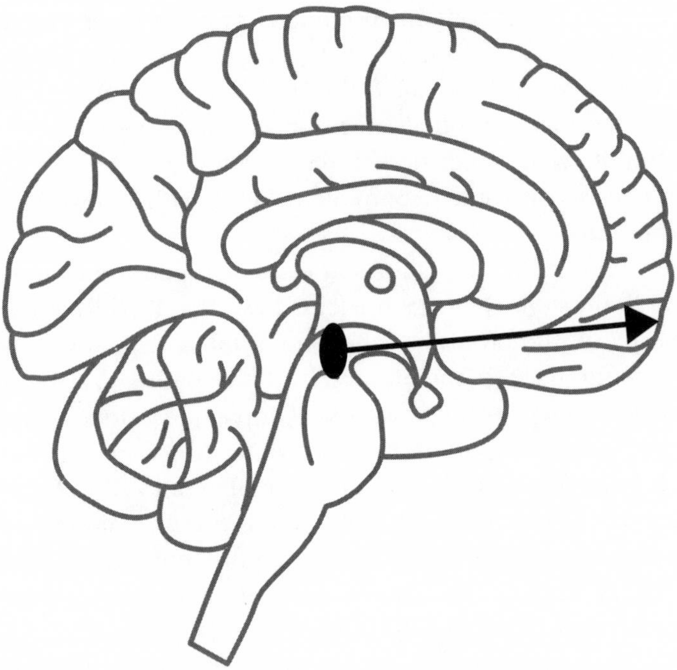

Figure 10.1. Schematic drawing of the ventral tegmental area and the reticulofrontal pathway damaged in Kevin's case.

we were able to do for him. Our treatments worked to a point, and a slight but quantitatively demonstrable improvement did take place. But the old Kevin was gone and we could not bring him back. We tried very hard to help restore Kevin's shattered executive functions, but our success was modest at best. Yet by giving us the opportunity to observe and describe the reticulofrontal disconnection syndrome, Kevin helped us, through his personal catastrophe, to better understand the workings of the frontal lobes. This understanding, in turn, sheds light on many disorders affecting the frontal lobes.

Kevin's condition was unusual, and highly informative, in yet another respect. His was the first well-documented case of remote memory impairment without a comparably severe deficit of new learning (retrograde amnesia without anterograde amnesia). In this respect he also enriched our understanding of the brain mechanisms of memory. But this is a separate story told elsewhere.[3]

Schizophrenia: A Connection That Was Never Made

Schizophrenia is a devastating disorder of the mind that affects approximately 1% of the population. It is at least in part a hereditary disorder, but environmental factors play an important role in its clinical expression and course. Schizophrenia seems to be more prevalent, and has an earlier onset, in males than females. The first overt manifestations of schizophrenia usually take place in the late teens to early twenties. Hallucinations (mostly auditory, "hearing voices") and delusions set in. They are usually paranoid, threatening in nature. The psychotic episodes are intermittent, interspersed with periods of relative mental health.[4]

But in addition to the psychosis, schizophrenia is characterized by a cognitive deficit, which is permanent, present even between the psychotic episodes, and is often even more debilitating than psychosis. Two early students of schizophrenia, Emil Kraepelin and Eugen Bleuler, were well aware of this, as is reflected in the original term for schizophrenia, *dementia praecox*, or "early loss of mind." The functions of the frontal lobes are particularly disrupted in schizophrenia. In his classic book, *Dementia Praecox and Paraphrenia* Kraepelin, wrote:

> On various grounds it is easy to believe that the frontal cortex, which is especially well developed in man, stands in close relation to his higher intellectual abilities, and these are the faculties which in our patients suffer profound loss in contrast to memory and acquired capabilities. The manifold volitional and motor disorder . . . makes us think of finer disorders in the neighborhood of the precentral convolution. On the other hand, the peculiar speech disorders resembling sensory aphasia and the auditory hallucinations . . . probably point to the temporal lobe being involved. We must imagine that the speech disorder is more complicated and less circumscribed than is sensory aphasia. The auditory hallucinations, which exhibit predominantly speech content, we must probably interpret as irritative phenomena in the temporal lobe.[5]

Contemporary neuropsychological and neuroimaging methods highlight the severity of frontal lobe dysfunction in schizophrenia. Of all the neuropsychological tests, schizophrenic performance is particularly impaired on the Wisconsin Card Sorting Test (WCST).[6] Since patients with frontal lobe damage find the WCST particularly vexing,[7] this is taken as evidence of frontal lobe dysfunction in schizophrenia.

Even more direct evidence of frontal lobe dysfunction in schizophrenia has been provided by the methods of functional neuroimaging. In healthy people the frontal lobes are usually more physiologically active than the rest of the cortex.[8] Neuroscientists refer to his pattern as "hyperfrontality." Hyperfrontality in normal individuals is a robust, highly replicable phenomenon, which does not depend on the method of neuroimaging used. It can be demonstrated with electroencephalography (EEG), positron emission tomography (PET), and single photon emission computerized tomography (SPECT).

In certain disorders, however, the pattern of hyperfrontality disappears. It is replaced with "hypofrontality," which means that the frontal lobe activity deteriorates relative to other parts of the cortex. Hypofrontality is a sure sign of severe frontal lobe dysfunction. Daniel Weinberger and his colleagues at the National Institute of Mental Health used PET to study brain activation patterns in schizophrenia. And true enough, severe hypofrontality was revealed.[9]

Popular conceptions of schizophrenia emphasize hallucinations and delusions, the so-called positive symptoms. But mental health professionals increasingly realize that the "negative" symptoms are far more debilitating. The negative symptoms of schizophrenia are the telltale symptoms of frontal lobe dysfunction. They include lack of initiative and drive and affective flatness. Schizophrenic patients tend to perseverate, which we know by now to be a frontal symptom. They are notorious for "loose" and "tangential associations," which are remarkably akin to the field-dependent behavior common in frontal lobe damage. Just think of Vladimir's monologues.

The first overt psychotic manifestation of schizophrenia usually takes place at about the age of 17 or 18. Eighteen is also the age of the functional maturation of the frontal lobes. Is this coincidental? Probably not. It is possible that the organism is able to compensate for a faulty development of the frontal lobes to a point. But once the disparity between the required adaptive frontal lobe function and its actual limited contribution hampered by disease reaches a certain point, the whole system decompensates and clinical disorder becomes evident.

Why are the frontal lobes particularly affected in schizophrenia? This question leads to a broader question. What is the cause of schizophrenic disorder? The puzzle is far from solved, but some of the pieces are already in place. Beginning at the turn of the twentieth century, various treatments have tried to cure schizophrenia without much success. Some of these treatments were, in retrospect, pretty horrific: shaking therapy, fever-inducing animal blood and syphilis-infected blood transfusion, and insulin coma among them.[10] Finally, in the 1960s a class of medications was introduced which appeared to have a genuine therapeutic effect. These "neuroleptics" acted on the neurotransmitter dopamine (DA). Neuroleptics were quite successful in reducing the so-called positive symptoms of schizophrenia: hallucinations and delusions.

The discovery of neuroleptics marked a turning point not only in treatment of schizophrenia, but also in the understanding of its mechanisms. The reasoning followed a simple syllogism. Neuroleptics relieve psychotic symptoms in schizophrenia. Neuroleptics act on the dopamine system. Therefore, schizophrenia is a disorder of the dopamine system. The logic behind this argument is patently flawed. According to this logic, an accident victim in a wheelchair had lost a pair of wheels, not a pair of legs. Drug efficacy does not always mean that the drug acts directly on a disordered ingredient.

Yet despite the logical flaw behind its rise to prominence, the dopamine theory of schizophrenia, has taken hold and received support from other experimental sources. Today it is widely accepted that the dopamine system is somehow impaired in schizophrenia, either by itself or as a consequence of a mismatch in the way dopamine interacts with other neurotransmitters, such as γ-aminobutyric acid (GABA) and glutamate.[11] But which dopamine system? Several are known to exist in the brain. Of particular interest to us are the nigrostriatal and mesolimbic–mesocortical dopamine systems.

Both systems originate in the brain stem, the nigrostriatal DA system in the nucleus called *substantia nigra* and the mesolimbic–mesocortical DA system in the *ventral tegmental area.*[12] The nigrostriatal dopamine pathway projects into the basal ganglia, a group of nuclei found below the frontal lobes, which are important for the regulation of movements. This pathway is not affected by schizophrenia itself, but it may be affected by the drugs used to treat schizophrenia.

The current thinking about schizophrenia focuses on the mesolimbic–mesocortical dopamine system. As I mentioned earlier, the disorder is presumed either to originate within this system or to be expressed through it as the remote effect of a disorder affecting glutamate, GABA, or other neurotransmitters.[13] The system diverges into two components: mesolimbic and mesocortical. The mesolimbic dopamine pathway projects into the deep (mesial) aspect of the temporal lobe. The mesocortical dopamine pathway is already familiar to us. It is the pathway that is disrupted in the reticulofrontal disconnection syndrome and which was presumably damaged in the fallen horseman. Dysfunction within this pathway probably also accounts for much of frontal lobe dysfunction in schizophrenia.[14]

Of course, the analogy between a schizophrenic patient and the fallen horseman is limited. In Kevin, the mesolimbic–mesocortical dopamine system had functioned properly up to the age of 36, when it was destroyed as a result of head injury. Kevin's cognitive development had completed its normal course before the injury. By contrast, in a schizophrenic patient the deficit is presumed to be neurodevelopmental. The mesocortical dopamine pathway fails to develop properly from the outset, due to some combination of genetic and environmental factors. This means that in schizophrenics the whole cognitive development is likely to be subtly different from that of healthy people. The cognitive development is abnormal from the beginning, long before the first overt clinical symptoms of schizophrenia are recognized. In Kevin the lesion was structural, caused by mechanical impact to the head. In schizophrenia the deficit is biochemical.

Yet despite the obvious differences between the two conditions, the neuroanatomy of the deficit is somewhat similar, in both cases affecting the projections from the ventral tegmental brain stem into the frontal lobes. Frontal disconnection appears to be central to both disorders, neurodevelopmental in one case, acquired in the other.

Abnormal dopamine biochemistry is probably not the only factor behind the frontal lobe dysfunction in schizophrenia. Fine quantitative CAT and magnetic resonance imaging (MRI) studies of schizophrenic brain revealed numerous structural abnormalities as well, including the decrement of the gray matter cortical volume.[15] The gray matter decrement is quite widespread and does not appear to be limited to any particular part of the brain. Still, some studies suggest that it is particularly pronounced in the frontal lobes.[16]

To conclude, both biochemical and structural factors may play a role in frontal lobe dysfunction in schizophrenia. Whatever the exact mechanisms of this dysfunction are, Kraepelin's prescient conclusion has been confirmed by modern neuroscience. Schizophrenia is to a large extent a frontal lobe disease.

Head Trauma: A Broken Connection

Traumatic brain injury (TBI) is a particularly poignant condition, since it is largely a disease of young people. In the beginning and middle of the twentieth century, traumatic brain injury involved mostly penetrating gunshot wounds. But in the Western world today TBI is usually caused by car accidents and job-related accidents. In the popular lore traumatic brain injury lacks the drama of Alzheimer's disease, acquired immunodeficiency syndrome (AIDS), or schizophrenia, but it is an epidemic of similar proportions. Since in the United States more than 2,000,000 people sustain TBI annually, it is sometimes referred to as the "silent epidemic."[17]

In the majority of cases, the so-called mild head injury, a seemingly complete recovery occurs within a few weeks of the injury. There is no lasting loss of movement, language, or perception. Deficit of memory and attention may persist longer, but eventually they also disappear. These patients are pronounced "fully recovered" and sent off to enjoy life.

Yet in subtle ways these young people are no longer their own selves. Drive, initiative, and competitive edge are often gone. They become passive and indifferent. Frequently they become inappropriately jocular, emotionally volatile, irritable, fractious, and impulsive. To an ordinary observer, these changes usually do not signal neurological impairment. In the tradition of naive dualism, they are often dismissed as "personality changes," as if "personality" were an extracranial trait. But in fact these changes reflect subtle impairment of the executive functions, subtle dysfunction of the frontal lobes.

The CAT and MRI scans are usually normal in these patients. For years, this contributed to the belief that the patients did not suffer lasting brain damage. Indeed, in most of these patients there is no structural lesion *within* the frontal lobes. But with the advent of functional neuroimaging, it became possible to study the physiology of the frontal lobes, in addition to the structure. Joseph Masdeu and his colleagues used SPECT to study brain blood flow patterns in mild head trauma patients.[18] Invariably, blood flow was abnormal, and often it was reduced in the frontal lobes. This pattern of "hypofrontality" was present even when the MRI scan was normal.

Like schizophrenia, closed head injury presents a puzzling picture of frontal lobe dysfunction without a frontal lobe lesion. And again, the mechanism is likely to be damage to the projections from the brain stem into the frontal lobes—the reticulofrontal disconnection syndrome. Neurologists have always felt that such damage is likely to occur in head injury. Today it is finally possible to understand both its causes and its consequences.

The news emanating from this understanding is both good and bad. The bad news is that the prevalence of lasting impairment following even "mild" head trauma is higher than had been thought. Almost invariably, the impairment affects frontal lobe functions. The good news is that identifying the cause is the first step toward developing effective therapies. The effects of reticulofrontal disconnection are presynaptic. Since there is no lesion *within* frontal lobes, the receptors for the critical neurotransmitters (the chemicals in charge of signal passage between neurons) are largely intact.

This opens the door for truly "cognotropic" pharmacology in closed head injury.[19] By cognotropic I mean the kind of pharmacology that is directed specifically at the cognitive deficit. There is nothing new about giving medications to patients recovering from head injury. However, the traditional rationale behind these treatments was directed at the control of seizures, depression, or other common consequences of head injury, but not at the cognitive deficit itself. It was not until the mid-1990s that the first attempts were made to use pharmacology directly to improve cognition of patients recovering from traumatic brain injury. Not surprisingly, in light of the previous discussion, this pharmacology targets mostly the dopamine system.[20]

Attention Deficit/Hyperactivity Disorder: A Fragile Connection

If one were to run a "disease of the decade" contest, attention deficit disorder (ADD) and attention deficit/hyperactivity disorder (ADHD) would be among the plausible contenders.[21] At the close of the twentieth century and the beginning of the twenty-first, the diagnosis is made generously and casually, often with little understanding of the underlying mechanisms, and sometimes with none at all. Parents actively seek the ADD diagnosis for their children to explain their school failures, and adults seek it for themselves to explain their life failures. It is not uncommon for a patient to ask the doctor "to diagnose my ADD." The proposition, of course, is utterly oxymoronic, about as sensible as asking: "What is the color of my green sweater?" But many doctors oblige, and those who do not often run the risk of losing their patients to those who do (it happened to me). It is not unheard of for a patient to shop for a doctor until the magic diagnosis is obtained.

When a diagnosis is not merely suffered but sought, clearly we have more than a clinical disorder. We have a social phenomenon. Why ADD has become a social phenomenon may well be worth a separate sociological and cultural anthropological treatise. I believe that it has to do with a complex combination of several cultural factors.

First, it has to do with the guilt, parental or personal, for one's child's or one's own failures. A clinical diagnosis removes the guilt and even the sense of responsibility. In an age when diagnostic labels proliferate, this offers a convenient way of unburdening the responsibility for life's failure. Second, it has to do with the ever-expanding scope of the individual rights and antidiscrimination concept. A clinical diagnosis earns all kinds of concessions and exemptions in wide-ranging situations. Third, the ADD phenomenon is true to the indefatigable American belief that anything can be fixed with the right pill (in this case, Ritalin). This may explain why another heavily inflated diagnosis of our time, learning disability (LD), is nonetheless nowhere nearly as commonly made or sought after: there is no ready promise of a magic pill.

Finally, the general public appeal of the ADD diagnosis has much to do with the illusory transparency of the very notion of "attention." Just as with "memory," everyone has an immediate, albeit often misguided, sense of the word's meaning. This, in turn, leads to an equally misguided sense of confidence in one's self-diagnosis. After all, nobody has introspection into one's pancreas, but everybody has introspection into one's own mind. As a result, very few lay individuals would presume to make the self-diagnosis of pancreatitis, but most people would have no compunction self-diagnosing their ADD.

Together with verbal and nonverbal learning disabilities of various stripes, and probably even more so, ADHD is among the more elastic diagnoses even when made by qualified professionals. This is inevitable, given that ADHD is a syndrome not linked to any single, well-defined pathogen. Disorders caused by distinct pathogens can be thought of in inherently discrete terms. Any notion of "continuity" between hepatitis B and hepatitis C would strike an infectious disease expert as nonsensical. But syndromes defined as constellations of cognitive symptoms are inherently idiosyncratic. This is particularly so when the syndromes in question may be caused by a number of different pathologies. And this is further complicated when all these pathologies have broad and overlapping ranges of neuroanatomical expressions. Since the pattern of cognitive deficit depends more on the neuroanatomy of the disorder than on its biological cause (a circumstance that many physicians and psychologists fail to fully grasp), the relationship among cognition, neuroanatomy, and the biological cause of the disease becomes particularly complicated. As a result, cognitively and behaviorally constructed syndromes should be thought of not as intrinsically discrete entities but as regions on continuous multidimensional symptom distributions with inherently arbitrary borders.

The additional complication, both conceptual and practical diagnostic, is that the pathological processes that produce the neurodevelopmental disorders in question are almost never focal, since mother nature is under no obligation to adhere to our discrete taxonomic manuals. This leads to the so-called comorbidity of different learning disabilities and ADHD, which is really not comorbidity at all, since the different syndromes in question seen in combination in a single individual are usually all caused by a single, albeit neuroanatomically distributed, pathological process rather than separate pathological processes.

With such a cluttered background, it is important to restore some measure of precision to the terms "attention" and "attention deficit." Attention deficit/hyperactivity disorder is a genuine and highly prevalent condition, which can be rigorously diagnosed and treated. Attention has often been compared to a flashlight illuminating a certain aspect of our mental or physical world against the background of competing distractors. Is there any biological reality behind the flashlight metaphor? There just may be. As we explore the analogy, we will see that attention involves complex neural machinery consisting of the prefrontal cortex and its connections.

Once we link ADHD to frontal lobe dysfunction, its very high prevalence (even when the diagnosis is made rigorously and conservatively) should come as no surprise. As we already know, frontal lobes are particularly vulnerable in a very broad range of disorders, hence the very high rate of frontal lobe dysfunction. The diagnosis of ADD or ADHD commonly refers to any condition characterized by mild dysfunction of the frontal lobes and related pathways in the absence of any other, comparably severe dysfunction. Given the high rate of frontal lobe dysfunction due to a variety of causes, the prevalence of genuine ADHD should be expected to be very high. But saying merely that ADHD is a mild form of the frontal lobe disorder oversimplifies the matter.

To pursue the flashlight analogy further, let us remind ourselves that a flashlight is an instrument. Someone (or something) must be responsible for choosing the direction in which it is pointed and for maintaining a steady hand. In neural terms, this means that the goal of action must be identified and it must effectively guide behavior for a period of time. We already know that goal-setting and goal-maintenance are provided by the *prefrontal cortex.* This is the actor whose hand controls the flashlight.

The flashlight analogy also implies the stage in need of illumination. The stage is found in the brain mostly in the *posterior aspects of the cortical hemispheres.* These are the structures most directly involved in processing the incoming information. Depending on the goal at hand, distinct, particular parts of the posterior cortex must be brought into the state of optimal activation (illuminated by the flashlight, so to speak). The selection of these areas is accomplished by the prefrontal cortex, which directs the flashlight accordingly.

The flashlight itself is found in the nuclei of the *ventral brain stem,* which can selectively activate vast cortical regions through their ascending projections. The prefrontal cortex guides the "flashlight" through its own descending pathways into the ventral brain stem. Finally, the prefrontal cortex *modifies* its control over the flashlight, based on the *feedback* it receives from the posterior cortex.

In sum, attention can best be described as a looplike process involving complex interactions among the prefrontal cortex, ventral brain stem, and posterior cortex (Fig. 10.2). Breakdown anywhere along this loop may interfere with attention, thus producing a form

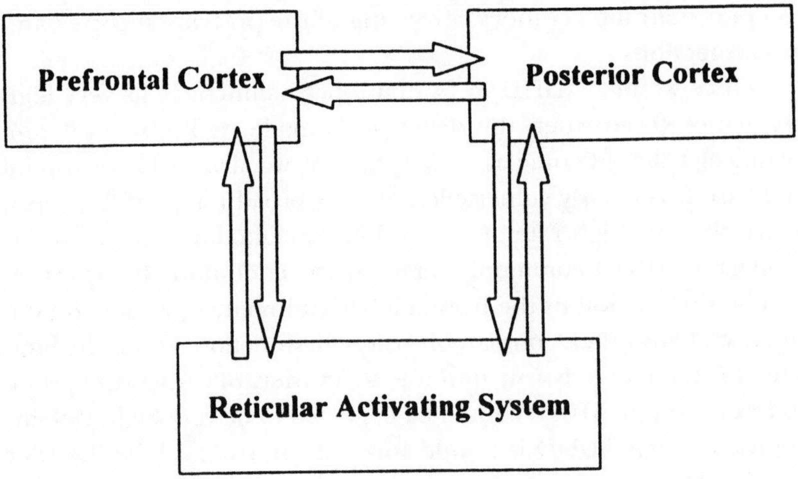

Figure 10.2. Frontal–reticular–posterior cortical attention loop.

of attention deficit disorder. The first consequence of the foregoing analysis is that the deficit of attention is among the most common consequences of brain damage. The second consequence of the foregoing analysis is that a number of distinct variants of attention deficit disorder exist, some with and others without hyperactivity.

The prefrontal cortex and its connections to the ventral brain stem (the hand holding the flashlight) play a particularly important role in the mechanisms of attention. When we talk about attention deficit disorder we usually implicate these systems. The exact causes of damage to these systems vary. They may be inherited or acquired early in life. They may be biochemical or structural. It should come as no surprise that the features of ADD are usually combined with some aspects of executive deficit. When the executive deficit is severe, the diagnosis of ADD becomes superfluous. But when it is mild, when the attentional impairment stands out and the executive deficit is minimal, then the diagnosis of ADD is properly made. In most such cases biochemical disorder affecting the frontal lobe connections is present, but there is no actual structural damage to the frontal lobes. In some cases the attentional deficit is highly encapsulated and may coexist with supreme capacity for planning and foresight. Winston Churchill may have been a case in point. Numerous descriptions of his behavior are strongly evocative of ADHD. Yet he was the man who foresaw the danger of Lenin, then Stalin, then Hitler, then Stalin again ahead of most other political leaders of the free world, and thus he can hardly be faulted for a lack of foresight.

Attention deficit in ADD is often selective. It is present only in the "uninteresting" activities but is absent in "interesting" activities. If the patient enjoys the task (a computer game or sporting event) and derives pleasure from it, his attention is on the mark. But attention drifts on any task devoid of instant reward, such as listening to a lecture or reading a textbook. This observation clearly links ADD to frontal lobe dysfunction. You will recall the role of the prefrontal cortex in goal-setting, volition, and delayed gratification.

The attention deficit disorder comes in a variety of forms. You will recall that the prefrontal cortex is functionally diverse (left–right; dorsolateral–orbitofrontal). Different anatomical patterns of frontal lobe dysfunction will disrupt attention in different ways. The pathways connecting the prefrontal cortex with the ventral brain stem nuclei are biochemically complex. Damage to different biochemical components within these pathways will also disrupt attention in different ways.

The "H" between the "D's" is the case in point. It is common to distinguish between attention deficit disorder (ADD) and attention deficit hyperactivity disorder (ADHD). It may very well be that the *hyperactive* form is most commonly associated with subtle dysfunction of orbitofrontal cortex and its pathways. This is why ADHD is often associated with the volatility of affect commonly seen in orbitofrontal damage. By contrast, the *nonhyperactive* form is more likely to be associated with subtle dysfunction of dorsolateral cortex and its pathways.

The distinction between ADD and ADHD is only the beginning. Numerous forms of attention deficit probably exist, requiring different remedies. As we learn more about the frontal lobes and their connections, we will be able to identify these forms and their remedies with growing precision.

ADHD Conquered: How Toby from Down Under Reclaimed Himself

Toby likes to say that he is an anomaly by definition, since he consists of three halves: half black, half Jewish, and half gay. Toby uses the word "black" generically, referring to all people of color, and the "half" in question is really not African but Polynesian. Nonetheless, all three "halves" represent minorities persecuted in many societies, with Toby at the intercept. And this is only the prelude to Toby's story.

Toby was adopted at the age of six days, so his exact background is unknown. Based on the information from his adoptive parents and his own research, his biological father was a French Jew and his biological mother was a Maori from New Zealand. They were college students in Sydney, and Toby was the obviously unwanted product of a date rape. His adoptive parents were a middle-class Welsh couple who immigrated to Australia from Great Britain. They wanted a daughter but adopted Toby because their older child (also adopted) was a boy and they did not have a separate room for a girl. This background of "unwantedness" had haunted Toby all his life, and he talked about it movingly in a documentary made about him many years later. The documentary, entitled *Alias*, was shown to critical acclaim at several film festivals in Australia, including the Bondi Film Festival and Sydney Short Film Festival (both in 1998).

Toby was a precocious child. He studied voice, the flute, and dance. Singled out for his exceptional talent, he performed solo at various gala events. But Toby was also a difficult, willful child. On many occasions, when his parents clashed with Toby, they practiced "tough love." They would pack a little bag with Toby's possessions and tell him to get out of the house and return only when he "repented."

Predictably, Toby would walk around the block and return knocking at the door, "repentant," until the next time. But once, at the age of nine, Toby did not return. Instead, he walked several miles in the middle of the night, clutching his little bag, from the suburb where he grew up to downtown Sydney. There he joined other homeless children and began his life as a street urchin.

For several years Toby was making a living as a hustler, a male street prostitute. Many years later he took me on a tour of "his" Sydney and brought me to the "Wailing Wall," a yellow sandstone structure, the exterior of Sydney's first jail off Oxford Street next to St. Vincent's Hospice, where the child hustlers used to congregate waiting for "johns." At first, I found my Jewish sensibilities offended by this sacrilegious reference, but then I acceded to its bitter accuracy. On the Wall, Toby showed me a faded graffiti "Toby, 1976," made during his life on the streets.

For all the other cases in this book I use fictitious names to protect my patients' confidentiality. "Toby", however, is in a sense a real name. It is one of several "noms de guerre" used by Toby in his profession as a child "sex worker" on the streets of Sydney. All these years Toby has been visiting his graffiti periodically, spending some silent time with it and making sure that it had not faded or been erased. He invited me to join him on this pilgrimage to his Wall, and I chose not to pry into the complex emotions that must have surrounded the ritual, and just stood silently by.

In the course of his street life Toby became addicted to numerous drugs—heroin, cocaine, speed, barbiturates, and anything else that he could find. Feeling increasingly desperate and trapped, Toby wrote this poem, "My Love for my Lady Sin," at the age of 16, likening his drug addiction to "Lady Sin":

A tale of sadness was born
In my love for my Lady Sin.
A story of trouble and woe,
And loneliness found within.

My lady stepped into my life
One night when I was alone,
And in the void she found in my heart
She quietly made her home.

The first year was fantasy, fiction.
The second a gay carousel.
By the third, the signs started showing,
By the fourth, my friends all could tell.

But still I worshipped my lady,
And one day I made her my wife.
And in my woe, with words "I do,"
I quietly gave up my life.

So my body and soul are now twisted,
That which did not waste away.
And I cry as I quietly remember,
It's the price we all have to pay.

This devotion doth turn to obsession,
My body as torn as my heart.
But still to my ear she whispers,
"Till death do us part."[22]

Then, at the age of 19, Toby sought out his adoptive parents, made peace with them, and embarked on an effort to rejoin the mainstream. Over the next few years he learned several trades. At various points he worked as a horticulture and hydroponics specialist, a nurse practitioner, a hairdresser, a makeup designer, a counselor for homeless children. By all accounts, he became quite accomplished in each of these trades. The only graduate with perfect test scores in the history of his agricultural college, Toby was invited to teach at the college immediately upon graduation, an unprecedented appointment. Faced with students often much older than himself and looking even younger than he was, Toby grew a beard to look "professorial." Toby was also becoming increasingly interested in creative writing and photography, and his work was beginning to meet with modest success. He had an amazing knowledge of animals and plants, and he used to maintain a menagerie consisting of several dogs, lizards, birds, and mice, as well as fish and frogs in the pond of the little Japanese garden he created in front of his house in a suburb of Sydney.

Despite his obvious and numerous talents, however, Toby was unable to hold a job. Sooner or later (usually sooner) Toby would get into violent arguments with his co-workers and end up fired or he would quit in a huff. He was restless and could not stick with any one activity. His adoptive parents hoped that Toby would take advantage of his obvious talent and become a veterinarian. But just as he was unable to settle in a job, Toby was unable to settle on a profession. The restlessness was pervasive and it played itself out in numerous ways. Toby attributed this restlessness to being multitalented, but it was clearly maladaptive.

Toby's personal relationships were also volatile and tumultuous, and his social persona was full of contradictions. He was known to be warm, loyal, and generous, someone who would never turn away a friend in need. At the same time he was explosive, quarrelsome, and belligerent even with his closest friends. He had a daughter out of wedlock and acted the part of a caring, devoted, and involved father, yet he was unable to settle into a marriage or any other sort of long-term relationship. When he finally did, the relationship was punctuated with volatility and outright violence, yet it was characterized by strong mutual commitment. He continued to fight his drug addiction, joined a methadone clinic, and finally, after several setbacks, was able to kick the habit.

I first met Toby during one of my frequent visits to Sydney, and then again when he visited New York. He was now in his thirties and full of contradictions. Immediately, Toby struck me as uncommonly intelligent and articulate, yet also uncommonly immature. Without actually having measured his IQ, I would guess it to be somewhere around 140–150, within a "very superior" range. Yet he was constantly caught unprepared for the consequences of his own and other people's actions, apparently unable to anticipate them. Things tended to constantly "happen" to Toby "all of a sudden," suggesting a glaring lack of foresight. Toby possessed an amazing amount of knowledge on an amazingly broad range of subjects, yet it was haphazard and unsystematic. At the same time, Toby was capable of an uncanny insight into people and situations at hand, and he was an exceptionally keen judge of human character. It appeared that his weakness of judgment was limited to the temporal domain, when some projection into the future was required. Toby was the most striking example in my personal experience of how noninterchangeable "insight" and "foresight" are, and how sharply divided these two abilities could be in the same individual. Toby was a man with superb capacity for *insight* and virtually zero *foresight.*

Restlessness was the dominant feature of Toby's personality, and it was evident in every interaction. The pressure to act, to move on, was palpable. He had a dozen competing plans and thoughts at any given time, all tripping over one another. In a group social setting, he had to talk with everyone simultaneously and then rush out in the middle of the dinner to do something else. A telephone conversation was invariably and suddenly interrupted in half-sentence with "I have to run." He had a volatile temper, with precipitous oscillations between gregarious charm one moment and brooding hostility the next. As I observed Toby's interactions with other people, I found his outbursts disturbing—extreme, unprovoked, almost frightening. Yet he was so obviously intelligent and gifted. He knew Sydney like the palm of his hand and was an insightful and witty guide.

Increasingly, I was getting the impression that Toby's outrageous behaviors had a life of their own, that Toby was engaged in them *in spite of himself,* and that he was in pain. As a result, my sympathy for Toby overrode my irritation at his antics. It was this combination of intelligence and pain that I connected with, and it made Toby attractive despite his very unattractive traits. Toby seemed to engender this reaction in other people too. He was, on balance, well liked and had many friends of all ages and from every walk of life who let him get away with behaviors not usually forgiven.

The clinician in me became more and more intrigued by what I saw. Toby was clearly hyperactive and also possibly suffered from a bipolar disorder. His affect fluctuated constantly and wildly. On a few occasions Toby made allusions to "highs" and "lows," confirming my observations. That Toby's life consisted of extreme states with very little in between was reflected in the diary he kept, true to his literary bent. The diary notes were entered from both ends of a big book: the "day section" and the "night section," referring to Toby's high and low points. In this context, Toby's past drug history looked like a desperate attempt at self-medication, a phenomenon not uncommon in people with subtle, undiagnosed conditions. I felt that I should talk to Toby and urge him to seek professional help, but an occasion did not present itself and I left Sydney without having this conversation.

I returned to Australia half a year later and Toby joined me for dinner at the Russian Accent restaurant in Sydney's Darlinghurst section. He did seem different. As if reading my mind, Toby started the conversation by recounting the events of the past few months. On his own, Toby had reached the conclusion that something was clinically wrong with him and that he was in need of professional help. He found a psychiatrist who put him on Dexedrine, a stimulant in the amphetamine family often prescribed to treat ADHD.

Dexedrine worked. Toby remained on it throughout my six-week stint as a visiting professor at the University of Sydney, and I was able to observe its effects on several social occasions (which included a visit to the Wailing Wall). Toby was calmer, more thoughtful, less argumentative, and no longer visibly hyperactive. There were no racing, competing, or conflicting ideas and no impulsive changes of mind every five minutes. There was no rush from one activity to another. Toby was able to sit and relax through a dinner, something he had not been able to do before; and now it was usually I who finished our telephone conversations with "I have to go." His affect no longer bounced from one extreme to another and was most of the time where it should be, at a pleasant, neutral level. For the first time since I had known Toby, he was predictable in a normal kind of way. Toby's capacity for organized, goal-oriented behavior had clearly improved as well. He no longer projected the image of immaturity and was talking and acting in a way that was, well, mature.

As I found out later, three months into treatment Toby developed depression, a known side effect of Dexedrine. He was switched to lithium but felt "lifeless," his "thought processes slowed down." With his doctor's consent, Toby decided to go completely off medications. Instead, he joined a support group and sought supportive psychotherapy. He feels that finally understanding his condition gives him power over it, and he is, on the whole, a much happier man. As of this writing, Toby continues to do reasonably well. He seems to have conquered his demons and successfully reclaimed himself.

For the first time in his life, Toby has been able to pursue things in a relatively systematic and methodical way. He bought a farm and is in the process of turning it into a thriving horticultural business. For the first time in his life he is making a considerable, steady income. At the end of my last visit to Australia, Toby showed up with a half dozen bottles of my favorite Australian reds, mostly Shiraz blends, as a parting gift. The wines were young and had to mature for four or five years, and Toby made a point of bringing this to my attention. "Could *you* delay gratification for so long?" I asked. "Now I could," came the answer.

As a friend, I was delighted to witness Toby's success. As a professional, I found it instructive that hyperactivity and attention deficit were so closely interwoven in this exceptionally bright individual with the textbook features of orbitofrontal dysfunction: poor planning and foresight, combined with diminished impulse control and exaggerated affective volatility. I could also place Toby's past drug addiction into a different perspective. It is not uncommon for people with various biochemical imbalances to self-medicate, usually with self-defeating results (although, admittedly, there were many factors in Toby's life on the street that may have contributed to his multiple addictions). And then, with successful treatment, these symptoms disappeared, or at least receded, in concert. Although we do not fully understand how Dexedrine (or, for that matter, Ritalin, Adderall, or other stimulants used to treat ADHD) works, it somehow helped strengthen the fragile frontal lobe connections to other parts of the brain.

Toby's life continues to be a struggle, stretches of success interspersed with painful reversals. The problem has not disappeared, but he has learned how to manage it, at least to a degree. The knowledge that his problem is biochemical helps Toby cope with it and removes the guilt and the shame. He no longer perceives it as a personal failure of character, but merely as a medical condition. Toby has learned to cope and to prevail.

Jerky Tics and Ticky Jokes

Frontal lobes are particularly closely linked with subcortical nuclei called the basal ganglia, especially with the caudate nuclei. This functional relationship is so close that the term "greater frontal lobes" may be warranted, by analogy with "greater New York," which includes Westchester, parts of Long Island, parts of Connecticut, and so on. Dysfunction within the frontal caudate system results in one of the most fascinating neurological conditions, Tourette's syndrome.[23] Tourette's is a fascinating disorder associated, among other symptoms, with involuntary motor tics and involuntary verbalizations, often highly inappropriate and offensive. It is precisely this provocative productive quality that makes it so intriguing.

Our culture traditionally approaches a neurological disorder as a deficit, a loss. This is reflected in our terminology: aphasia—loss of language; amnesia—loss of memory. Hypermnesia and hyperverbality, when they occur, are viewed by society as a mnemonic or literary gift, not as pathology. But if the norm is defined as the population average, then talent is, by definition, a deviation from the norm. The relationship between talent and psychopathology has intrigued and beguiled both clinicians and those afflicted (or blessed). Edgar Allan Poe, himself suffering from episodes of confusion, paranoia, and possibly seizures, wrote poignantly about genius and madness intertwined.[24]

It is common to distinguish in neurological and neuropsychological conditions between "negative" and "positive" symptoms. Negative symptoms reflect the loss of something that should normally be present, such as the ability to walk, talk, and see things. Positive symptoms reflect the presence of something that is not part of normal cognition, such as hallucinations or tics. Negative symptoms are more readily comprehensible, easier to conceptualize, measure, quantify, and subject to rigorous scientific examination. Positive symptoms are usually more elusive, more mysterious but also more intriguing and challenging. They hint at an inner world that is different and not merely impoverished—at the presence of a neurological condition which not only robs but also endows.

The link between creativity and mental illness is strikingly apparent in the lives and genius of van Gogh, Nijinsky, and Rimbaud. This is true also for some leaders with a particularly visionary brand of leadership, who shaped the history of our civilization in a way that suggests an exceptionally powerful "executive talent." Alexander the Great of Macedon, Julius Caesar, Peter the Great of Russia, and possibly Akhenaton (the Egyptian pharaoh who founded the first known monotheistic religion in the history of human civilization) suffered from epileptic seizures. Peaks of creativity and productivity were interspersed with nadirs of despair and mental paralysis in the lives and work of Byron, Tennyson, and Schumann, all of whom suffered from the bipolar manic-depressive disorder. On a more ordinary plane, I have often felt that the more gifted people in my personal surroundings paid a price for their talent in other areas of their mental life, and that the balance between gift and deficit is ruled by some unforgiving zero-sum equation.

If talent tends to come at a price, then certain neurological and psychiatric conditions may sometimes bring their own rewards. These conditions remain the source of fascination and intellectual challenge. Among such conditions, Tourette's syndrome is particularly intriguing and remains a source of fascination for scientists and the general public alike.

What makes Tourette's so intriguing is the richness and variety of positive symptoms associated with it. Originally described by George Gilles de la Tourette in 1885, this condition is characterized by uncontrollable facial and bodily tics, compulsive grunting vocalizations, profane verbalizations, and incessant exploration of the environment. These symptoms appear in various combinations, which often change over time. They may be subtle and masked or highly conspicuous. In the latter case they are often perceived as offensive and asocial.

Clinical observers of Tourette's patients also note a particular quickness of wit reminiscent of a fencing match and a peculiar cognitive style. Over the years of observing people with Tourette's, I came to recognize a unique and unmistakable mental quirkiness, quickness, and jerkiness of their thought processes. There are also peculiarly wicked, singularly irreverent and risqué, jousting flashes of humor. At the height of the Bill Clinton–Monica Lewinsky scandal a tourettic acquaintance of mine appeared, accompanied by his girlfriend, at a party in the house of a mutual friend and announced with a flourish: "Neither I nor my girlfriend had sex with the president." As a visual metaphor of tourettic cognition, Balinese dance comes to mind. This quick quirkiness of the mind goes hand in hand with the quick quirkiness of the movements. This is not all curse: some Tourette's patients are known to be gifted in sports like karate and basketball despite their condition.

The symptoms of Tourette's usually appear in childhood, sometimes triggered by a traumatic event, and often disappear with age. However, in many cases the symptoms persist through the life span. Tourette's tends to afflict males more often than females.[25] Because of the diversity of manifestations, it is increasingly common to talk about the "Tourette's spectrum" rather than a single Tourette's.[26]

Tourette's syndrome affects the neurotransmitter dopamine, which is one of the major biochemical systems in the brain, and neuroanatomical structures called the caudate nuclei, critical for the initiation of movements and more complex behaviors. In many cases Tourette's seems to have a hereditary basis. Anecdotally, Tourette's syndrome and Parkinson's disease (both disorders of the nigrostriatal dopamine system) sometimes run in the same families.

Some scientists believe that in Tourette's syndrome the caudate nuclei (one of the major basal ganglia) somehow escape from the control normally exerted over them by the prefrontal cortex. Together with the thalamus, the basal ganglia can be thought of as the evolutionary antecedents of the neocortex. In the course of evolution their original role was superseded by the frontal cortex, which in developed mammals exerts an inhibitory influence over the caudate nuclei. It appears that in humans the caudate nuclei trigger certain behaviors and that the frontal cortex puts these behaviors through a complex system of cognitive filters, "permitting" some of them and curtailing others.

I also believe that in Tourette's syndrome the moderating influence of the frontal cortex on the caudate nuclei is weakened. As a result of this disinhibition, peculiar behaviors arise, bearing a distinct similarity to frontal lobe syndromes. These behaviors are often so socially provocative that the patients are met with derision, ostracism, and sometimes even with physical assault.

The most provocative among them is coprolalia, from the Greek words "copra" for "feces" and "lalia" for "utterance." The patient makes profane exclamations in socially inappropriate situations.

Many years ago I salvaged from a likely arrest a decently dressed young man who was walking up and down a line of passengers (myself among them) waiting to board an Amtrak train at the 30th Street Station in Philadelphia and cursing us out in the foulest conceivable language. He was also exhibiting characteristic motor tics, which I immediately recognized as tourettic. As the cops were about to converge on him, I approached one of them and quickly explained what was going on. The officer listened and I was thankful to see him merely tell the man to get lost.

But coprolalia is not the only form of the characteristic tourettic "verbal incontinence." To understand the nature of this incontinence, we must again consider a loss of inhibition, which we discussed in connection with the orbitofrontal syndrome. At times we all have thoughts which social norms prevent us from voicing in public. Walking down the street I may note to myself in passing that someone is "fat," someone else is "ugly," and someone else again looks "dumb." I am able to contain these thoughts and they do not leave the sanctum of my cranium, so to speak. Not so with a Tourette's patient. What is on his mind may immediately be also on his lips. It may be unflattering epithets, slurs of various kinds, obnoxious editorial comments—anything forbidden. "Forbidden" seems to be the key to understanding the particular inability of some tourettic patients to contain the unprintable lexicon.

This brings up an interesting psycholinguistic question. Why would a language contain words that are culturally forbidden from being uttered? This sounds like an oxymoronic feature of the language. Yet as far as I know, most, and most likely all, languages contain such "forbidden" lexicon. It could be that they serve the function of emotional release, and it is precisely the act of discarding the barrier of prohibition that accomplishes the release. Forbidden fruit is sweeter! It seems that in Tourette's the urge to release internal tension may be ever present and unquenchable.

As we learn more about Tourette's, different subtypes of this disorder begin to emerge, which may reflect different patterns of the aberrant interaction between the basal ganglia and the frontal lobes. Oliver Sacks talks about the duality of Tourette's symptoms: "stereotypic" and "phantasmagoric."[27] These symptoms clearly parallel the two most conspicuous features of "afrontal" cognition, which we discussed earlier in the book: perseveration and field-dependency. In most cases of Tourette's, stereotypic and phantasmagoric symptoms do not appear in isolation but are combined in tourettic behavior in various proportions.

I believe that the relative severity of these symptoms reflects the relative involvement of the left or right caudate nuclei in any individual case. In many patients both symptoms are present, reflecting the bilateral nature of the disorder. However, relatively pure cases also exist, suggesting the existence of relatively lateralized caudate dysfunction. On the whole, the stereotypic symptoms seem to predominate, probably due to a particularly close relationship between dopamine and the left hemisphere.

Tourette's syndrome is often associated with obsessive-compulsive disorder (OCD) and attention deficit disorder (ADD). In OCD, repetitive behaviors dominate the patient's life, frequently in an extremely disruptive way. Obsessive behaviors resemble perseveration; in fact, they are perseveration. By contrast, ADD is characterized by extreme distractibility, often with equally devastating consequences for cognition. This distractibility is, in fact, a mild form of field-dependent behavior. I suspect that Tourette's is accompanied by the symptoms of obsessive-compulsive disorder when the left caudate nucleus is particularly involved. And it is accompanied by the symptoms of attention deficit disorder when the right caudate nucleus is particularly involved.

The stereotypic aspects of Tourette's take the form of forced repetitive behaviors, like motor tics and grunting vocalizations. These behaviors can be extremely conspicuous, branding the patient as "weird," a social pariah. The tics are often perceived as intentional grimacing and taunting. A friend of mine who developed symptoms of Tourette's at the age of five recalls being chased away from the playground by other children's mothers because they thought he was deliberately teasing them with his "grimaces."

The phantasmagoric symptoms are often expressed as an excessive (and often grotesquely so) urge to explore every incidental object in the environment. These symptoms are less common than the stereotypic, but they can be equally conspicuous. I was particularly struck by them many years ago, as I was walking on Manhattan's Upper West Side with Oliver Sacks, who has always been interested in Tourette's syndrome, and a tourettic friend of Oliver's by the name of S.F., an extremely intelligent and articulate man, then in his early thirties. The young man's exploratory behavior was extreme and he was drawn to everything in his path: a tree, an iron gridwork, a trash can. As we were walking down the street, he bounced from object to object, checking them out with all his senses. He looked, listened, touched, smelled, and licked them with his tongue. The whole spectacle was so bizarre that I turned to Oliver at some point and said: "I hope you have a picture ID on you, in case we all get arrested!" When we walked into a neighborhood restaurant, the young man immediately felt up the owner, an upright-looking middle-aged woman from Germany, under the scandalized stares of other guests. This was done with casual innocence, in passing. Since I was a customer, the German lady laughed it away and let it go, instead of throwing us out of her establishment or calling the police.

But it is not always easy to categorize a tourettic behavior as clearly stereotypic or clearly phantasmagoric. Often it appears as both. My friend Lowell Handler is an acclaimed photographer, filmmaker, and author, with an award-winning film, *Twitch and Shout,* and a book of the same title to his credit.[28] He has a relatively mild form of Tourette's. No matter whom he is talking to, several times in the course of the conversation Lowell will make a jerky fencing movement touching the other person with his hand and immediately withdrawing it. His friends are so used to this touching behavior that they ignore it completely. But it raises eyebrows and creates tensions with strangers. Is Lowell's urge to touch an exploratory behavior? Is it a perseveration? Or is it both?

I asked Lowell and S.F. to give an insider's view of their unusual urges and behaviors. This is what they said.

EG: You often have an urge to touch an object or a human being. What goes through your head at the moment and right before?

LH: It is heightened sensory curiosity and lack of inhibition. I become focused on a body part or an object. Once I focus on it, the urge becomes uncontrollable. It is an urge that I cannot resist.

SF: It is tactile curiosity, an urge to explore. I am attracted to a leather chair, plastic surface, or some other object that I must touch. It may take extreme forms. I once gagged on a toothbrush because I wanted to swallow it to find out what it feels like in my mouth. When I eat I sometimes have an urge to put my face in the food to feel the texture. Sometimes I have an

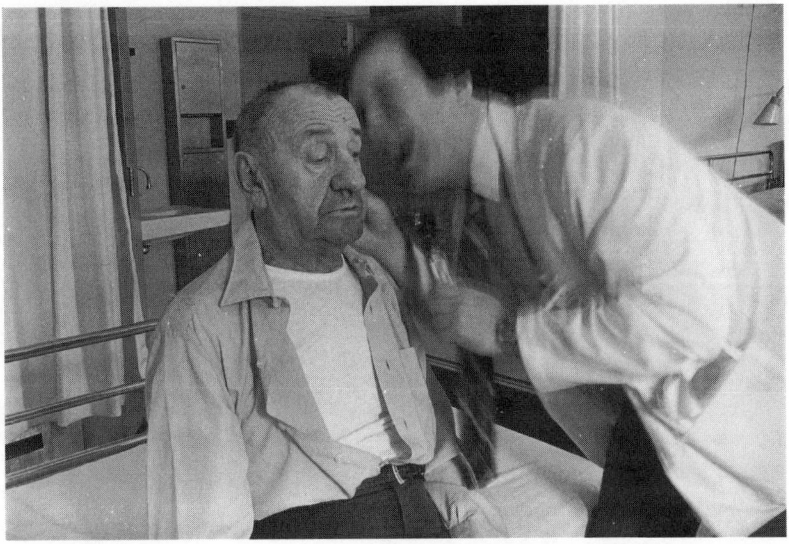

A

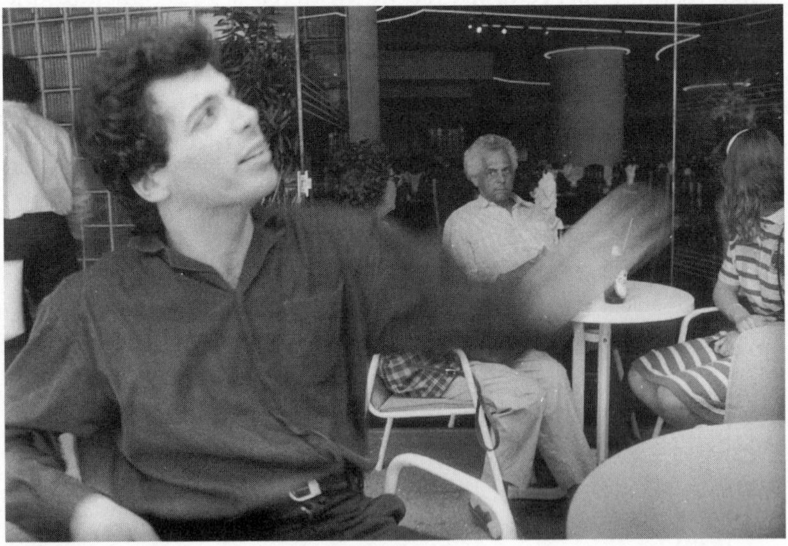

B

Figure 10.3. The art of Lowell Handler. Pictures of people with Tourette's taken by a photographer with Tourette's. (A) Ticking on the job. A doctor with Tourette's examines a patient with dementia. (B) Drawing glances. S.F. in a sidewalk café. (Reprinted with the photographer's permission.)

urge to probe the roof of my mouth with utensils like a knife and a fork until it bleeds. This is why I like to eat sandwiches, to stay away from the utensils, because even though it does not happen every time, sooner or later it will happen. I often eat with my hands; I don't care what people think. I can do it elegantly.

EG: Suppose the object of your interest is out of your reach. Would you climb over things to get it?

LH: I will be able to inhibit the urge, but Shane may not be.

SF: Sometimes when I see an object which I cannot touch at the moment I come back hours later to touch it. A few times I had an urge to touch things as I was moving heavy furniture. So I would balance the furniture with one hand and touch with the other.

EG: How extreme is this urge? Would you touch an object or a human even knowing full well that it may lead to destructive consequences? Or will you be able to inhibit the urge?

LH: I will probably be able to inhibit the urge.

SF: I constantly touch light bulbs and burn my fingers.

EG: Why the light bulbs?

SF: Because they are particularly shiny.

EG: How about people? Will you touch a cop on the street if you have the urge?

LH: I might touch his nightstick (laughs).

SF: I try to avoid places where I am surrounded with people, like the subway. Sometimes I would imitate a person instead of touching him.

EG: Is this urge to explore limited to the tactile sensations? Or does it involve other senses?

LH: It involves all of the senses. But for me it inevitably ends up being tactile.

SF: Also taste and smell. I sometimes used to put my face into the toilet bowl to taste the water. I do not do it anymore.

EG: What do you experience before and at the time of a tic?

LH: Sometimes there is a precursor to a tic, sometimes a quasi-sensation, like an "itch for a twitch." There is often a tension going through my body.

EG: As I am talking to Shane, I hear these barking sounds at almost regular intervals. Tell me more about this urge to vocalize (part of the interview was conducted over the phone).

SF: I am drawn to mimicking sounds. Sometimes I mimic animals, or some odd sounds idiosyncratic to particular people. I imitate them for hours, can't get rid of them. Sometimes I imitate fragments of a word. And sometimes the word doesn't suit me, but even when it is not "native" to me, I will still repeat it. If I listen to you long enough, I will incorporate your way of speaking into my own . . . probably not your accent but your verbal mannerisms.

EG: I can see that you are hypersensitive to sound. You keep interrupting me and asking me about every background street noise that reaches you over the phone.

SF: This hypersensitivity is true not just for noises but also for speech. I often adopt other people's stereotypic phrases and postures . . . I once read Constantine Stanislavski about imitation leading to a metamorphosis in an actor . . . when somebody else's mannerisms become yours . . . something like that. When I used to spend a lot of time with Oliver Sacks I adopted some of his mannerisms.

EG: Did he notice that?

SF: I don't think so.

EG: So your extreme sensory curiosity is tactile and gustatory and auditory in nature. How about visual? And how synthetic, or synesthetic, does it all get?

SF: All the senses play a role together. When I walk down the hall I want to feel everything, like a cold wall. I will pick the mood of it. I want to see left side and right side simultaneously. I want to wear the environment like clothes. I experience the disappearance of a person behind me like physical weight removed. When I move from a big room to a small room, I feel physical change like pulsating light.

LH: It is very visual with me also. I am incredibly visually oriented by what I do because I am a photographer. I am influenced by visual things and I am tempted by them.

EG: How about coprolalia? Why do some people with Tourette's have the urge to use profanities?

LH: Fuck you . . . That was a joke . . . Because it is forbidden. Tourette's is a lack of inhibition.

SF: I have this urge only to a very limited degree. I understand that only 12–14% of people with Tourette's develop strange phrases. With me it is not coprolalia, but saying things without feeling inhibited.

EG: If it is the lack of ability to inhibit forbidden thoughts, then how about other inappropriate utterances? If you see a fat person on the street will you say "fat," or if you see an ugly person will you say "ugly"?

LH: I won't but some people with Tourette's may. I knew a woman with coprolalia. We went to a very upscale Manhattan restaurant together, and as we were talking she would shout something derogatory about every person who walked in. Two gay guys were sitting next to us and she said "faggots," a black guy was sitting nearby and she said "nigger"; two guys with pony tales walked in and she said "hippies." This was not directed only at others; she was making derogatory comments about herself and me, too. She said "My family are . . . spicks," and "you Lowell are a . . . kike." Then we finished lunch and walked down Eighth Avenue and somebody bald walked by and she shouted out "baldie." She was trying to inhibit these slurs but they were very audible.

SF: No, I won't make slurs, but I may do a pantomime, like I may have a barely perceptible movement in my belly to imitate an extended belly when I see a fat person on the street.

EG: Does your Tourette's affect your mental processes also? Is there such a thing as a "tourettic cognitive style" or "tourettic personality"?

LH: Tourette's produces a higher-order lack of inhibition. This makes it difficult to concentrate, makes me very distractible. There is a low frustration threshold in Tourette's. I used to slam things into walls, break and smash things. I also think that my irreverent sense of humor is part of my Tourette's. I was once at a party and someone said that he was gay. To which I said that I was trisexual: males, females, and animals.

SF: Increased risk taking is part of Tourette's. I once stopped when I saw a man mugging a little girl and intervened.

EG: Some doctors working with Tourette's believe that Tourette's is associated with hypersexuality. What to do say to that?

LH: I consider myself hypersexual and think it is part of my Tourette's. But to me hypersexuality is just a special case of being generally hypersensitized to any experience. In sex you deal with a sensory enhancer and Tourette's enhances attraction to everything.

SF: In this culture everything is sexualized, but I do have huge energy and wide tastes, certainly for a 40 year old.

EG: Does Tourette's make your life difficult?

LH: Yes, because of the stigma. Ignorant people misconstrue the symptoms and try to explain them within their own limited frame of reference. Once somebody asked me if I was dancing. On another occasion somebody told me to shut up.

SF: Tourette's does make my life difficult, less because of the tics and other symptoms themselves and more because of social issues. The social issues easily eclipse Tourette's itself. I had violence directed at me at college, at the karate school. In addition to assaults I have been arrested many times, once while visiting my father in the hospital, while they were looking for someone else. I was suspected of rape for no good reason. I have been harassed by cops for doing nothing, just for ticking . . . A man once tried to push me off the subway platform. I did not call the police, because I did not think police would believe me because of my tics. And some time later the same man pushed a girl under a train . . . And I felt bad about not reporting him earlier . . . But not all cops are like that. There are some very enlightened cops.

EG: Does Tourette's add anything positive to your life?

LH: Definitely, but it takes a certain talent to turn it into an asset. The compulsions and obsessions of Tourette's give me an edge in getting work done, in bringing things to a closure. There is a compulsion to complete work, to go an extra step. Tourette's makes me hypersensitive, it gives me sensory curiosity, really a multisensory curiosity. This is important in writing and photography. It gives me an extrasensory component, it sensitizes me, clues me into things. My inner world is richer because of this.

SF: Now I know that it does. A higher degree of athletic ability is common in Tourette's. The sense of smell is very acute. I once smelled freshly cut grass far from the place where it was being cut, way before anyone else could smell it. People with Tourette's are much more inquisitive than other people . . . Tourette's gives you a great sense of humor . . . Tourette's gives you energy, but it is merciless.

EG: How does Tourette's affect your relationships with other people?

LH: It sort of scans out certain people who would not be interested in me anyway. So I am left with the people to whom to my Tourette's does not matter. And these are the people I want to be with.

SF: I lost a few friends, but I was able to help other people. When I worked in a summer camp, I once saw a boy, 17–18 years of age, who could not stop washing his hands. He had an extreme case of obsessive-compulsive disorder. He was washing his hands for literally an hour and could not stop. I was the only one who understood what was going on. I turned off the faucet, gently dried his hands with a towel, and escorted him out of the bathroom.

EG: How does Tourette's affect your identity?

LH: My identity is definitely one of a touretter. There is a Tourette's culture of being on the outside and I have a sense of brotherhood with other outsiders. I feel closer to other frowned-upon groups of people with differences of all kinds. I feel that they have a better insight into my condition.

SF: Tourette's is one of my identities, but not the only one . . . By the way, I dislike the word "touretter." It demeans the condition, makes it sound like a vocation.

EG: There is a certain popular mystique about Tourette's syndrome. How do you explain it?

LH: There is that mystique and I have become a poster boy for Tourette's. Tourette's has a mystique and a cult both glamorized and tainted with infamy. Tourette's is a disability and is off and odd, yet it resonates with our culture of overabundance. Unlike other disorders, Tourette's is not something shortchanged with life, but something overloaded with life. In these times of extreme political correctness and prudishness people tip their hat to us, because we are full of life, intoxicated with it.

SF: One should differentiate between mystique and mystery. What people usually see is a panoply of odd things that have been exploited in movies to dramatize things, often in a way which has nothing to do with the substance of the character or the reality of Tourette's.

EG: Is your Tourette's the defining fact of your life?

LH: It definitely is for me.

SF: Socially, yes to a major extent. Privately less so. My life is not just unidimensional.

EG: How do you cope with your Tourette's?

LH: I try to ration myself a certain amount of quiet time alone in my apartment. An occasional drink helps . . . and a lot of vitamins.

11

"What Can You Do for Me?"

"Cognotropic" Drugs

For many neuropsychologists, like myself, science is a labor of love, but seeing patients is bread and butter. Traditionally, the clinical contribution of neuropsychology has been mostly diagnostic, with precious little to offer patients by way of treatment. Neuropsychology is not the only clinical discipline for years consigned to helpless voyeurism. Every discipline concerned with cognition shares this humbling predicament. A psychiatrist treating a schizophrenic patient or a depressed patient finds himself in a similar position. He has ample pharmacological tools to treat the patient's psychosis or mood, but very little to treat the patient's cognition. Even though psychiatrists increasingly recognize that cognitive impairment is often more debilitating in their patients than psychosis or mood disorder, traditionally very little direct effort has been aimed at improving cognition.

A neurologist treating a patient recovering from the effects of head injury does not fare much better. He has adequate means to control the patient's seizures but not his cognitive changes, despite the fact that cognitive impairment is usually far more debilitating than an occasional seizure. Society had been so preoccupied with saving lives, treating hallucinations, controlling seizures, and lifting depression that cognition (memory, attention, planning, problem solving) had been largely ignored. Granted, various neuroleptics, anticonvulsants, antidepressants, sedatives, and stimulants do have an effect on cognition, but it is an ancillary effect of a drug designed to treat something else.

Alzheimer's disease and other dementias have been society's wake-up call. Here, in the most affluent country in the most affluent of times, human minds were succumbing to decay before human bodies, a sharp challenge to the tacit popular belief that "body is frail but soul is forever." This provided an impetus for the development of an entirely new class of drugs, which can be termed familially as "cognotropic." Their primary and explicit purpose is to improve cognition.

Since medical and public preoccupation with dementia focuses on memory, most of the pharmacological efforts have been directed at improving memory. At the time of this writing, a handful of drugs known as "Alzheimer's drugs" or "memory enhancers" have been approved by the Food and Drug Administration. In reality, both designations are somewhat misleading. The drugs in question are anti-cholinesterases. They are designed to inhibit an enzyme necessary for the breakdown of the neurotransmitter acetylcholine in the synapse, and thus to prolong its action after its release into the synapse. Acetylcholine is a neurotransmitter which plays an important role in memory as well as in other cognitive functions. Biochemical processes involving acetylcholine ("cholinergic transmission") are impaired in Alzheimer's dementia, but they are also impaired in many other disorders.

In fact, my first encounter with this class of drugs took place in the late 1970s and involved physostigmine (Antilirium), a first-generation anticholinesterase, now out of use as a cognitive enhancer. We gave it to a patient recovering from severe head injury.[1] The problem with physostigmine was that its length of action (half-life) was so miserably short that no sustained therapeutic effect could be reasonably expected. At best, a very fleeting, short-term improvement could be hoped for. To capture this fleeting improvement, my colleagues and I designed a brief battery of neuropsychological tests, which my research assistants Bob Bilder and Carl Sirio rushed to administer with clockwork timing during carefully calculated, and very narrow, windows of opportunity. But fleeting though it was (and at times overshadowed by vicious diarrhea), subtle memory improvement was reproducibly present. This was a cause for hope that with some improvements this class of medications could someday have real clinical value.

A number of years later, tacrine (Cognex) appeared on the market, followed by donepezil (Aricept). These drugs are also anticholinesterases, but with a much longer action and a more meaningful therapeutic effect. They should not be thought of as exclusively "Alzheimer's drugs" since their utility is not limited to Alzheimer's disease. I have observed a significant, albeit transient, therapeutic effect of these drugs on cognition in patients with Parkinson's disease and brain damage due to hypoxia.

Although their effect is still transient and inconsistent, the advent of these second- and third-generation anticholinesterase drugs opened a new chapter in pharmacology, ushering in cognotropic medications. In the next few years we will undoubtedly witness a boom in the cognotropic pharmacology acting on various biochemical systems. Much further research is needed for it to become established and some controversy is inevitable, but the concept of cognotropic drugs is provocative and timely.

Interesting work on cognotropic pharmacology is being done in Europe as well. An audacious program to investigate neuroanatomically precise effects of various drugs has been under way in Russia for some time. Scientists at the Bourdenko Institute of Neurosurgery in Moscow, where I trained in Luria's lab 30 years ago, have reported an array of specific drug effects. According to them, levodopa (L-dopa), a precursor of the neurotransmitter dopamine, improves the functions we typically associate with the posterior aspect of left frontal lobe: motor sequencing, speech initiation, expressive language. To put it in technical terms, the Russians claim that L-dopa reduces the symptoms of dynamic aphasia, transcortical motor aphasia, and Broca's aphasia. By the same token L-dopa seems to retard the functions commonly associated with the parietal lobes (spatial orientation and spatial construction). L-Glutamic acid, an analogue of the neurotransmitter glutamate, improves, according to the Russians, other functions associated with the frontal lobes. It improves insight into one's condition (reduces symptoms of anosognosia), improves the sense of humor, time estimation, and time sequencing. L-Glutamic acid also improves the functions commonly associated with the parietal lobes. L-Tryptophan, a precursor of the neurotransmitter serotonin, improves the functions of the parietal lobe but retards the functions of the frontal lobes. At the same time, L-tryptophan interferes with the functions of the frontal lobes, particularly the left frontal lobe. Ameridin, an anticholinesterase not commonly known in the United States, seems to improve the functions of the parietal lobes, particularly the left parietal lobe. It improves comprehension of grammar and reduces the symptoms of "semantic aphasia."[2] These claims made by the Russian scientists associating various neuroactive drugs with particular cortical functions are more specific, and in a way more ambitious, than most Western claims to this effect. They require careful review and replication, but they are extremely provocative.

But where do the prefrontal cortex and the executive functions fit in? Executive deficit is easily as common and debilitating as memory impairment, and so there should be as much societal pressure for the development of cognotropic frontal lobe pharmacology. Here, too, developments are at an embryonic stage, but some forward movement is evident. We have discussed the role of dopamine in frontal lobe function, so it should come as no surprise that dopamine-enhancing pharmacology has shown some promise.

The dopamine system is complex, with a number of different receptors. To be truly effective, dopamine pharmacology must be receptor-specific. As we learn more about the variety of dopamine receptors, we are learning about the receptor-specific action of dopamine-enhancing drugs. Bromocriptine (Ergoset or Parlodel), a dopamine D2 receptor agonist, has been shown to improve working memory, a function closely linked to the frontal lobes, in normal adults.[3] The efficacy of two more recently developed D2 receptor agonists, ropinirole (Requip) and pramipexole (Mirapex), has yet to be established.[4]

Currently, a great deal of interest exists in identifying specific dopamine receptors and developing receptor-specific pharmacology. But the thrust of this research is driven by the treatment of schizophrenia, which requires dopamine receptor–specific antagonists. To boost the function of the frontal lobes, dopamine agonists may be required with an affinity to various dopamine receptors, including D1 and D4. This poses a new challenge to pharmaceutical industry and research.

Cognotropic pharmacology of the frontal lobes holds out particular promise in those disorders where frontal lobe dysfunction is present without massive structural damage to the frontal lobes. In such conditions neurotransmitter receptor sites are largely intact, which makes pharmacological intervention more promising. Mild traumatic brain injury (TBI) is such a condition. This is a particularly poignant disease, since it afflicts young people, often in good physical shape and with undiminished life expectancy. Following traumatic brain injury, problems with working memory, with decision making, with attention, with motivation, and with impulse control are common. Bromocriptine tends to improve these functions in the patients with head injury.[5] So does amantadine (Symmetrel), a drug presumed to facilitate dopamine release and delay dopamine reuptake following its release into the synapse.[6]

The advent of these drugs signals the beginning of "frontal-lobe cognotropic pharmacology", I hope with much more to follow. But the true excitement will come when the cutting-edge pharmacology is combined with the cutting-edge neuropsychology, when fine cognitive measures are used to guide cognotropic pharmacology in precise, individualized ways. The actor-centered cognitive tasks shown to be so exquisitely sensitive to distinct variants of frontal lobe dysfunction may prove to be particularly useful in guiding custom-tailored cognotropic pharmacology of the frontal lobes.

Jogging the Brain

In August 1994 I picked up a copy of *Life* magazine with a picture of human brain on the cover.[7] The article suggested that mental exercise may help forestall the onset of mental decline associated with aging. *Life* magazine is not where new ground in neuroscience is usually broken, and the idea sounded a bit sensational. But some of the world's top neuroscientists were interviewed for the feature and stood behind it. Among them were Arnold Scheibel, director of the prestigious Brain Research Institute of the University of California, Los Angeles; Antonio Damasio, director of the Neurology Department at the University of Iowa School of Medicine, the author of the best-selling *Descartes' Error* and *The Feeling of What Happens*;[8] Zaven Khachaturian, a leading scientist at the National Institute of Aging in Bethesda, Maryland; and Marilyn Albert of Boston's renowned Massachusetts General Hospital. A few years earlier the notion of cognitive exercise as a method of prevention of mental decline would have scandalized serious neuroscientists as snake oil. But now the tide was clearly changing.

I was thrilled with the *Life* magazine article because it resonated with my own intuition. As a clinical neuropsychologist, I have spent a significant part of my career studying the patterns of recovery from the effects of brain damage and designing cognitive rehabilitation methods. My mentor, Alexandr Romanovich Luria, was a pioneer of cognitive exercise as a way of spurring the recovery from the mental effects of brain damage, first developing this approach during World War II to help soldiers with head wounds. The neurologist and author Oliver Sacks, my friend and colleague, has written eloquently and poignantly about the therapeutic effects of mental stimulation on dementia of the elderly. My own experience has led me to conclude that cognitive stimulation can serve as a powerful catalyst for the natural recovery from the effects of traumatic brain damage.

Treatment and prevention often call for similar approaches. Vaccines developed to protect against infection with viral diseases such as hepatitis B have been shown to reduce clinical symptoms in those already infected. In the efforts to fight AIDS, some scientists, like Jonas Salk, believe that future vaccines will serve a dual function: they will protect healthy population and slow down the disease progression in those already infected with human immunodeficiency virus (HIV).

The idea of systematic cognitive exercise as a way of improving mental functions is not new. For decades, people who suffered head injury or stroke have been treated with cognitive therapy as a way of restoring mental functions lost to brain damage. Today we are on the threshold of a conceptual leap from treatment to prevention. A growing number of scientists, physicians, and psychologists believe that vigorous and diversified mental exercise may help in the battle against the decline of mental functions, which ultimately may take the form of dementia. From treatment to prevention: this is the dominant theme of modern medicine, and it is becoming an important theme in the battle against cognitive decline.

The theme has gained currency as the general public is made increasingly aware of the ravages of dementia. Earlier, mental deterioration was assumed to be a normal and inescapable product of aging. "Becoming sclerotic," "getting senile," "losing one's marbles" were the standard popular terms for referring to such "inevitability." But recent scientific research has shown that a large portion of the elderly population never loses mental acuity through gradual, inexorable decline. Instead, scientific research suggests a "bimodal" picture, a distinct difference between those who lose their cognitive powers with age and those who do not. In their influential book *Successful Aging*, John Rowe and Robert Kahn make the point with impressive clarity.[9] From this it follows that cognitive deterioration is not an obligatory part of *normal aging*. It is a *disease* of aging which affects some, perhaps many, but not all. The disease is called "dementia" and several types of dementia exist, each representing a different type of illnesses afflicting the brain. Therefore, we usually talk about "dementias" rather than "dementia."

A preordained, inexorable progression toward "senility" is a myth. This is the good news. The bad news is that while not inevitable, dementias are very common. Alzheimer's type dementia is the most common among them, accounting for more than 50% of all dementias. By the age of 65, more than 10% of the population is afflicted with one form of dementia or another. According to the American Medical Association, by the age of 85, some 35% to 45% of people have it to at least some degree. It is estimated that dementias are likely the fourth or fifth most common cause of death in the United States.[10]

The high rate of dementia means that something must be done to treat it, and preferably prevent it. Unfortunately, mental illness (and dementia is a form of mental illness) has been traditionally associated with stigma. People are more open about their "physical" ailments than they are about their "mental" ailments. Stigma means silence and the illusion of absence. Therefore, the taboo imposed by tradition on the discussion of mental illness has hindered society's ability to grasp its full scope and dimension and to assign the battle against it the priority it merits.

Fortunately, attitudes are rapidly changing. With the development of science and public awareness, the distinction between "physical" and "mental" ailments is becoming increasingly obsolete. Until recently, the general public was under the blissful assumption that while the body is frail and subject to decay, the mind is forever invulnerable. Today most people understand that the "mind" is a function of the brain, which is very much part of the "body."

The courageous statements by Ronald Reagan and other public personalities have lent the cause of dementia a sense of urgency and dignity. The growing popular awareness of dementias and an open discussion about this disease are welcome developments, aligning the public sense of priorities neatly with reality.

How can dementias be fought? Again, the thrust must be two-pronged: treatment and prevention. A concerted effort has been launched by scientists and the pharmaceutical industry to develop dementia-treating drugs. Little of immediate clinical utility has been accomplished, but the battle has been joined, the resources have been mobilized, and there is good reason for optimism in the long run. As was discussed in the previous section, several Alzheimer's-fighting medications have been approved, most of them targeting the cholinergic neurotransmitter system in the brain.

By contrast, the concept of prevention of cognitive decline is only beginning to take shape in the minds of the scientific community and has yet to enter the public consciousness. Over the last few decades, the concept of physical exercise as a way of extending one's physical well-being with age has taken a firm hold in American culture. Today, the notion of cognitive exercise as a way of extending one's cognitive well-being with age is becoming increasingly accepted by scientists and is beginning to connect with the public consciousness.

While the concern about cognitive decline and how to prevent it naturally increases with age, it need not be limited to the elderly. A certain decline of cognitive powers is already evident at the age that we usually associate with the zenith of our lives and the pinnacle of our careers: the forties, fifties, and sixties. A green youth is usually more adept at learning a foreign language, computer language, or a complex game like chess than is a corporate or political leader at the height of his or her power and societal influence. We begin to notice subtle memory slippage long before our confidence in ourselves becomes eroded in a global sense. Is this inevitable? Are our lives governed by a cruel Faustian deal, so that as we approach the pinnacle of our lives we lose something of ourselves?

Today a prominent professional or a powerful corporate leader refuses to accept as an inevitable fact of life the tradeoff between the success that comes with age and the loss of physical youthfulness. Physical exercise is viewed as a way of slowing down physical erosion of the flesh. Taking care of one's body enhances the way one is perceived, both professionally and socially; the opposite also occurs, as chain smoking and gluttony stigmatize one as a slob out of touch with modernity.

But ours is an "information age." The relative competitive importance of brain versus brawn has been reversed over the centuries and today success hinges more on brain than brawn. Corporate duels, political contests, and scientific rivalries are not fought hand to hand or toe to toe. They are fought brain to brain and mind to mind. In modern warfare, too, the sharpness of the minds is decisive, not the sharpness of the steel. The outcome of military conflicts is increasingly decided by technological and scientific sophistication.

Increasingly, the advent of new computational technologies, virtual reality, and the Internet will bring together the human nervous system and manmade computational devices in a fundamentally new interface. We will need our brain more than ever in the brainy new age. How can we protect it from disease and decline?

The body of information essential to the workings of society is increasing exponentially, and never in the course of human civilization has there been an informational explosion as rapid as today's. The history of human civilization can be described in terms of a ratio of the amount of knowledge added to the total knowledge bank by a given generation to the amount of knowledge inherited from the previous generation. In antiquity, this ratio was close to zero, the rate of knowledge accumulation was slow, and the curve was almost flat.

The rate of knowledge accumulation has shot up particularly in the last century, and it continues to increase. It is already true today that much of the knowledge that we acquire in school becomes obsolete by the time we reach our career peak. In the past, a university graduate could spend the bulk of a career complacently reaping the fruits of his or her early accomplishments. Today, large amounts of knowledge must be acquired throughout life in order to stay professionally afloat.

The slope of the information curve determines how different cultures place different premiums on the tradition embodied in the experience of the old as opposed to the innovation embodied in the daring of the young. The informationally static cultures of antiquity were built on a reverence for the old. Vestiges of this attitude are seen in the contemporary, but traditional, cultures of Asia and part of Europe. By contrast, American society, which among the major contemporary societies is the youngest and least rooted in tradition, is based on a reverence for youth. This is undoubtedly a reflection of its informational dynamism. The message contained in this analysis is clear: retaining mental vigor throughout life has never been as essential to success as today. It will get even more so!

The body of essential information is growing exponentially, but the human brain has remained biologically unchanged, or changed very little. It is commonly said that the computational capacity of the brain is virtually unlimited and can accommodate the body of knowledge of virtually infinite size. This common biological assumption is challenged by history. Whatever the theoretical computational capacity of the brain is, in a practical sense it proves to be limited. It was possible for an educated person of antiquity to be in command of virtually all the essential knowledge of the time. This is no longer possible. Around the High Middle Ages or Renaissance the body of essential knowledge in human culture exceeded the mental capacity of a single individual. Knowledge was becoming increasingly distributed and specialized. Paradoxically, the admired Renaissance man was the first human *not* capable of holding all the essential knowledge of the time. The ability to integrate diverse knowledge in an informationally fragmented world is clearly a decisive competitive advantage for those who can do it. This too calls for particular mental sharpness.

Middle-aged people engage in physical exercise to improve their odds against having a heart attack. Young people are unconcerned about this. They exercise for a totally different reason: to improve their social attractiveness. But the criteria of social attractiveness reflect the attributes critical for competitive success, which in turn change through the history of human civilization. The criteria of physical attractiveness reflect the markers of physical fitness, which has been, and will remain, an important ingredient of success. For centuries the definition of attractiveness has revolved mostly around physical attributes.

This is changing. We are entering an unprecedented era in the development of human society ruled overwhelmingly by information processing. Bill Gates refers to this as the advent of the knowledge-based society. As we move into the twenty-first century and beyond, the attributes of social attractiveness will reflect the prerequisites of success in the increasingly information-driven society. Sharp will be beautiful. Being perceived as "dumb" will be even more socially damning than being perceived as "ugly." In this social context, any credible approach to the preservation of cognitive wellbeing will be met with a public sense of approval and urgency.

History of Cognitive Rehabilitation

What can we learn from the experience of cognitive exercise as treatment to apply to the idea of cognitive exercise as prevention? The history of cognitive rehabilitation as a way of helping recovery from stroke and head injury is long, and the results are mixed. Several decades ago Alexandr Luria introduced the concept of a "functional system." Any complex behavior controlled by the brain as a whole, he reasoned, was a result of the interaction between a number of specific brain functions, each controlled by a particular part of the brain. He called such an interactive constellation of specific functions responsible for a complex mental product a functional system. The same cognitive task can be accomplished by different routes, each based on a slightly different functional system. The simple analogy with skilled movements helps illustrate the point. Most people lock the door with their right hand under most circumstances. However, if your right hand is occupied or injured, you should be able to do it with your left hand. If you need to lock the door while carrying two shopping bags, each in one hand, you can hold one bag with your teeth while quickly pulling the key and locking the door with the free hand.

What will happen to a functional system in brain damage? World War II was raging and Luria's mandate was to develop ways to help soldiers with head wounds recover their mental abilities. The brain damage is likely to affect only a few, but not all, the components of a functional system. The challenge, then, is to rearrange it so as to replace the impaired components with different, intact ones. The specific composition of the functional system will change but its overall product will not. A new functional system is introduced through retraining the patient in order to form a new cognitive strategy for the same mental product.

Although this sounded good in theory, the method did not always work in practice. The transfer of training was the stumbling block. Imagine the patient who lost his memory as a result of head injury. A common way to restore his functions was to teach the patient various strategies to memorize word lists of increasing length. In the end, the patient would become spectacularly successful in memorizing word lists, but what difference does this make in real life? The real-life outcomes of such training were mixed. There was little generalization from one specific use of memory to others. To me, the enterprise had the ring of politically driven Soviet "scholarship" to it; and I noted to myself that in private Luria talked about cognitive rehabilitation somewhat dismissively. By way a curious historical digression, politicized Soviet science was led by Trofim Denisovich Lysenko, a Stalin-era agronomist and barely literate neo-Lamarckian, who claimed that he had a method for making acquired traits hereditary. This was a typical, if extreme, exercise in "Marxist science" designed to exalt the miracle of Soviet agriculture. By contrast, genetics was declared "bourgeois pseudoscience" and banished. Of course there was no scientific basis behind Lysenko's claims. Meanwhile, genetics was retarded in Russia for many years, despite Russia's early lead in the field.

The relative lack of success of generalization in cognitive retraining is disappointing but not entirely surprising. Research has shown that the capacity for generalization in problem solving is limited even in neurologically healthy people. It is not as if they showed no generalization at all, but this generalization tends to be "local" rather than "global." People tend to learn by acquiring situation-specific mental templates.[11] It is only logical to assume that the capacity for generalization is even more limited following brain damage.

These considerations led to the rise of a more modest, concrete approach. Instead of attempting to help recover a mental function in a general, open-ended way, very specific, practical situations were identified in which the patient had difficulties. Training was then directed at these situations specifically, and narrowly. This approach worked, but by its very essence it was of inherently limited value. And it held little romantic appeal to the clinicians.

Brain Plasticity and Cognitive Exercise

These early efforts, with their mixed results, were based on the premise, or at least hope, that cognitive training helps change cognitive functions. The field changed radically with the new evidence that cognitive exercise helps change *the brain itself.* It seems almost self-evident that this should be the case. When you engage in an athletic activity, not only do your athletic skills improve, but actual muscle growth takes place. By contrast, lack of exercise leads not only to the loss of athletic skills, but to actual muscle tissue reduction. Of more immediate relevance, sensory deprivation of an infant monkey will produce an actual atrophy of the corresponding brain tissue.

The critical evidence, however, has begun to emerge only recently. It has been known that immersion into an enriched environment facilitates the recovery from the effects of brain damage in rats.[12] Now the mechanisms behind this recovery are finally becoming clear. The recovery of animals with traumatic brain injury was compared under two conditions: in an ordinary environment and in an environment enriched with an unusual amount of diverse sensory stimulation. When the brains of the two groups of animals were compared, striking differences were revealed. The regrowth of connections between the nerve cells ("dendritic sprouting") was much more vigorous in the stimulated group than in the ordinary group. There is also some evidence that with vigorous mental exercise, blood supply to the brain improves through enhanced growth of small blood vessels ("vascularization").[13] Scientists like Arnold Scheibel believe that similar processes take place in the human brain. Systematic cognitive activation may promote dendritic sprouting in the victims of stroke or head injury; this in turn facilitates the recovery of function.

This invites another question: Does cognitive activation slow down the progression of degenerative brain disorders, such as Alzheimer's disease, Pick's disease and cortical Lewy bodies disease? These disorders are characterized by progressive brain atrophy and loss of synaptic connectivity. This is associated with the accumulation of pathological microscopic entities, such as amyloid plaques and neurofibrillary tangles in Alzheimer's disease.

Unlike head trauma or stroke, dementias are slow, insidiously progressive disorders. This means that the efficacy of treatment should be judged not just by whether it reverses the course of the disease (this, for the time being at least, would be an unrealistic expectation) but also by whether the treatment slows the disease progression. Evidence exists, however, that for limited periods of time cognitive exercise can actually improve brain physiology, even in an absolute sense. Scientists at the Max Planck Institute in Germany used positron emission tomography (PET) to study the effects of cognitive exercise and neurostimulant medications on brain glucose metabolism in people at an early stage of cognitive decline. Administered together, the two treatments enhanced brain glucose metabolism.[14] The German study examined the changes of resting brain physiology, its background state, and also the changes in the pattern of brain activation when stimulated by a cognitive task. The advent of sophisticated brain-imaging technology gives us a window into the brain basis of mental processes, which would have been deemed unthinkable in the past. It is now possible to observe directly what happens in the brain as the person is engaged in a mental activity.

For years, the prevailing assumption among scientists was that the brain loses its plasticity and capacity for change as we move from childhood to adulthood. Today, however, new evidence is increasingly available that the brain retains plasticity well into adulthood and possibly throughout the life span. The earlier assumption was that in an adult organism dying neural cells could not be replaced. In fact, although there has long been evidence that new cells could develop in birds (owing to the work of the Rockefeller University scientist Fernando Nottebohm) and rats (owing to the work of Joseph Altman at the University of Indiana), it was dismissed as an exception rather than the rule. But recent work by Elizabeth Gould of Princeton University and Bruce McEwen of Rockefeller University has shown that neurons continue to divide in the adult marmoset monkey.[15]

Neural cell division was demonstrated in the hippocampus, the brain structure particularly involved in memory. In another study Elizabeth Gould and her colleagues found an ongoing proliferation of new neurons in the cortex of the adult macaque monkey.[16] The new neurons are added to the heteromodal association cortex of the prefrontal, inferior temporal, and posterior parietal regions, the brain areas involved in most complex aspects of information processing.

The new evidence, arising both from animal studies and from research with humans, opens an entirely new way of thinking about the effects of cognitive exercise. *Rather than attempting to shape or reshape specific mental processes, try to reshape the brain itself.*

While most of us agree that brain processes are mental processes, the logic behind the various approaches to cognitive retraining is different. Early efforts emphasized particular functions in the hope that the brain structures corresponding to that function would somehow be modified as a result. The new approach emphasizes generalized, open-ended effects of cognitive exercise on the brain. A tennis player or a golfer engaged in daily practice may aim at improving a particular stroke. This is akin to a specific task-oriented cognitive training. Or, he may hope that by practicing a few particular strokes, he will improve his other strokes and therefore the game as a whole. This is akin to functional system-based cognitive training. Or, finally, he may embark on an exercise regimen with the goal of improving not so much the game in and of itself but the body that plays it: to increase his strength, coordination, and stamina in a very general way. This is akin to trying to improve brain function. The third goal is far more ambitious than the first two, but new evidence suggests that it is attainable, at least in principle.

Animal studies show that improvement of "brain power" through cognitive activation is more than a fantasy. Scientists at the famed Salk Institute for Biological Studies in southern California examined the effects of enriched environment in adult mice.[17] They found that mice placed in cages filled with wheels, tunnels, and various toys developed up to 15% more neural cells than the mice left in standard cages. The "stimulated" mice also did better than their "unstimulated" counterparts on various tests of "mouse intelligence." They were able to learn mazes better and faster.

These findings are critical in two respects. First, they debunk the old notion that new neurons cannot develop in an adult brain—they can. Second, these findings demonstrate with dramatic clarity that cognitive enhancement may actually change brain structure and improve its information-processing capacity. The new cell growth was particularly evident in the dentate gyrus of the hippocampus, a structure on the mesial surface of the temporal lobe considered to be particularly important in memory.[18]

The emergence of new nerve cells ("neuronal proliferation") in the adult brain appears to be linked in the so-called neuroblasts, the precursors of neurons, which in turn develop out of generic cell "prefabricates" called the stem cells. The stem cells and neuroblasts continue to proliferate throughout adulthood, but usually they do not survive to become neurons. The Salk Institute study suggests that cognitive stimulation increases the neuroblasts' chance of survival to become full-fledged neurons.[19]

Among all the applications of cognitive exercise, its preventive role helping people to enjoy their cognitive health for the longest time possible is particularly exciting. Both anecdotal observations and formal research suggest that education confers a protective effect against dementia. Highly educated people are less likely to succumb to its effects. The MacArthur Foundation Research Network on Successful Aging sponsored a study of the predictors of cognitive change in older persons. Education emerged as by far the most powerful predictor of cognitive vigor in old age.[20]

The basis for this relationship is not fully understood. Does the life-style associated with education protect against dementia, or is it that some people are born with a particularly robust neurobiology, which makes them better candidates for advanced education and protects them against dementia? It is reasonable to assume that it is the nature of activities associated with advanced education that protects against dementia, rather than education itself. Highly educated people are more likely to engage in lifelong vigorous mental activities than less educated people due to the sheer nature of their occupations.

Assuming that neurological dementia-causing illness strikes both groups with equal frequency, then equally severe neurological illness will have a less disruptive effect on the well-conditioned brain than on the poorly conditioned brain. This will be due to the extra reserve that the well-conditioned brain has by way of additional neural connections and blood vessels. Equal amounts of structural damage will produce less functional disruption. Again, the analogy between cognitive conditioning and physical conditioning comes to mind. The case of Sister Mary makes the point with dramatic and remarkable clarity. She performed well on cognitive tests until her death at the age of 101. And this is despite the fact that the postmortem study of her brain revealed multiple neurofibrillary tangles and plaques, the hallmarks of Alzheimer's disease. It would appear that Sister Mary had an intact mind inside an Alzheimer's brain!

Sister Mary was one of the School Sisters of Notre Dame, the much-studied and reported nuns from Mankato, Minnesota. Remarkable for their longevity, they were also known for the absence of Alzheimer's disease among them. The phenomenon was unanimously attributed to the lifelong habit of being cognitively active. The nuns constantly challenged their minds with puzzles, card games, debates of current policy issues, and other mental activities. Furthermore, the nuns with college degrees, who taught and engaged in other mind-challenging activities on a systematic basis, on average lived longer than their less well-educated counterparts.[21] So compelling were the observations of the nuns' cognitive well-being that a postmortem brain study was designed to examine the relationship between cognitive stimulation and dendritic sprouting.

In the case of nuns, the protective effect of cognitive exercise on the brain appeared to be cumulative, extending over the whole life span. Old convent records were found, containing the nuns' autobiographies written when they had been in their twenties. When the relationship between the nuns' early life writings and the prevalence of dementia in later years was examined, a striking picture emerged. Those nuns who tended to write more grammatically complex and conceptually rich essays in their youth retained their mental vigor until much later in life than those who wrote simple factual prose as young women.[22]

These findings prompted speculation in the popular press that dementia is a lifelong process, which begins to subclinically affect some people early in life, causing them to write simpler prose. But it is just as likely that the aspects of brain organization that make some people "smarter" than others also confer a protective effect against later-life dementia. Then again, it is also possible that the nuns who developed the habit of taxing their minds early in life, and presumably kept the habit, acquired the protective effect on the brain which proved to be of critical importance in their advanced years.

Is the protective effect of prior cognitive stimulation on mental decline universal? It appears to be, since the effect can be demonstrated in other species as well. This was demonstrated by Dellu and colleagues in male Sprague-Dawley rats.[23] Animals with previous experience of learning various tasks were less susceptible to age-related memory deficits than the rats without the history of "mental exercise."

"Use it or lose it" is an old adage. It seems to apply to the mind directly and literally. Two scientists at the Pennsylvania State University, Warner Schaie and Sherry Willis, published a paper with the provocative title "Can Decline in Adult Intellectual Functioning Be Reversed?"[24] The authors studied a group of individuals, aged 64 to 95 years, who suffered cognitive decline in a variety of mental functions over a 14-year period. Could a relatively brief cognitive training regimen restore their mental performance to its original level, to compensate for 14 years of decline in spatial orientation and inductive reasoning? In many instances, the answer turned out to be "Yes." Furthermore, cognitive recovery was generalized; it could be demonstrated on several independent tests of the cognitive functions of interest, and not just on the procedures used for training. The effect was lasting; in many participants it could be demonstrated seven years after the completion of the training regimen. The authors concluded that the training regimen reactivated the cognitive skills, which had become "rusty" from lack of use.

If it is logical to expect the therapeutic effects of cognitive exercise, why did earlier attempts at cognitive rehabilitation of the effects of brain damage meet with such mixed success? There are several reasons. The first reason lies in the very difference between the cognitive retraining of a damaged brain and cognitive conditioning of an intact or almost intact brain, between treatment and prevention. Medical knowledge dictates that it is easier to prevent an illness than to treat it. A severely damaged brain is predictably less likely to respond to any kind of remedy than a basically healthy brain responds to prevention.

The second reason relates to how cognitive exercise has been traditionally designed under the "old" philosophy. In an attempt to target a specific, very narrow, cognitive function, targeted cognitive exercises were used. It is logical that the more broad-based a cognitive workout regimen, the more general the effects. To use a physical fitness analogy, an individual who spends all the exercise time on one machine cannot be expected to improve his or her cardiovascular system. For that one needs a diverse circuit.

The third reason relates to the ways the effects of treatment are measured. By measuring the effects of one cognitive exercise with the ability to perform on a different cognitive task, we are making an assumption about the specific nature of therapeutic effects that are being measured. Failure to find an effect may indeed result from the true lack of effect. But it may just as easily reflect our failure to find an appropriate measure to detect it. Since we are trying to enhance the underlying biological processes, it would be better to measure such processes directly. And indeed, when the effects of cognitive exercise were evaluated with positron emission tomography (PET), improved glucose metabolism (an important marker of brain function) was found.[25]

The fourth reason relates to what constitutes reasonable expectations of the effects of a cognitive workout. If general brain functions are enhanced through such conditioning, then the expected effect may be broad but subtle.

In any event, the recent findings of ongoing neural cell proliferation throughout the life span have breathed new life into the enterprise of cognitive exercise and endowed it with a new rationale.

Cognitive Fitness: Beginning of a Trend

The benefits of physical exercise are well known, but how to exercise is another matter. Some people do chin-ups on their kitchen door, and others go to a cardiovascular fitness center. While the chin-ups are probably good for you (unless, of course, you break the kitchen door), you stand to gain more from a sophisticated workout. This is why we spend time and money on exercise equipment, personal trainers, and health club membership fees.

A well-designed exercise circuit takes advantage of the knowledge of human anatomy and physiology. Each exercise is designed to enhance the function of a particular muscle group or physiological system. Depending on your individual goals, you may choose a complete, well-balanced circuit or focus on a particular exercise. The workout of a college athlete getting ready for a crew meet is not the same as the exercise of his overweight, middle-aged professor concerned with his cardiovascular system and trying to ward off a heart attack.

The brain is referred to as the microcosm for a reason. Of all the biological systems, it is the most complex and diverse in function and structure. The knowledge of the brain's exquisite complexity provides a sound basis for the design of a "brain exercise circuit." Here, a particular mental exercise is designed to match a distinct cognitive function. Most of us are vaguely aware of the benefits of cognitive challenge. As with physical fitness, your mental workout can be less or more sophisticated. Your Sunday morning crossword puzzle is probably good for you; think of it as the chin-ups for the mind. But you can do much better than that.

If cognitive exercise improves and enhances the brain itself, then it is important to design a systematic workout, ensuring that *all*, or at least *most*, of the important parts of the brain are engaged. In physical fitness training, it is important to exercise various muscle groups in a balanced way. Balance is achieved through workout circuits involving diverse and carefully selected exercises. Contemporary knowledge of the brain makes it possible to design a "cognitive workout circuit", that will systematically train various parts of the brain. If undirected—in effect random—mental exercise has a demonstrably protective effect against dementia, then a targeted, scientifically designed cognitive workout regimen should be even more beneficial.

Early symptoms of Alzheimer's disease and other primary degenerative dementias, such as Lewy bodies disease, are quite diverse. Memory decline, suggestive of hippocampal dysfunction, is the first sign of illness in most patients, but not in all. In some patients early decline is expressed as word-finding difficulties implicating the left temporal lobe; as spatial disorientation implicating the parietal lobes; or as the impairment of foresight, social judgment, and initiative—

signs of frontal lobe dysfunction. While in general all these areas are susceptible to the effects of Alzheimer's disease, their relative vulnerability appears to be highly variable. What determines the relative vulnerability of different brain structures in different individuals?

Scientists from the Netherlands Institute for Brain Research in Amsterdam, Mirmiran, van Someren, and Swaab, put forth a mind-boggling hypothesis.[26] They believe that the activation of selective brain areas throughout a lifetime may prevent or delay the degenerative effects in those parts of the brain. According to this view, someone engaged in design as a profession or hobby will protect his or her parietal lobe, someone engaged in creative writing will protect his or her temporal lobe, and someone engaged in complex decision making and planning will protect his or her frontal lobes.

British neuroscientists reported a finding that, even a few years earlier, would have been dismissed as a neurological impossibility. They scanned the brains of 16 London taxi drivers and compared them with the brains of 50 control subjects.[27] The taxi drivers, who in the course of their work develop an intricate mental map of their huge metropolis, had larger posterior hippocampi. Furthermore, the greater the number of years spent on the job, the larger the hippocampi were in individual drivers. Not surprisingly, the hippocampi are presumed to be involved in spatial learning and memory.[28] This may very well be the first direct demonstration of a relationship between the size of a brain region and the environmental factors contributing to its use.

The logical conclusion of this line of reasoning is provocative and striking. To protect the *whole brain* against the effects of diffuse degenerative disease, a *comprehensive cognitive fitness regimen* must be designed, engaging various parts of the brain in a balanced and scientifically grounded manner. The concept of systematic cognitive exercise as an important activity both in aging and during the peak career years is still new. But it is a natural and logical extension of physical exercise. "Physical fitness" has become a household term. *Cognitive fitness* is on its way to becoming the next trend in popular culture.

Beginnings of a Program

My clinical practice of neuropsychology is quite diverse. A significant part of it involves bright and intelligent aging men and women who have lived full and successful lives. Many of them are retired professionals (scientists, doctors, book editors) who have lived by their minds, enjoyed the powers of their minds, and are now concerned by a subtle cognitive decline. Sometimes a neuropsychological evaluation will confirm their concerns and sometimes it won't. But our diagnostic instruments are relatively crude and a very subtle cognitive change may remain unnoticed. When an obviously intelligent patient reports the impression of mild decline, I tend to believe the patient more than the numbers generated by my tests.

Patients all come for a diagnosis, but even more so, they come for help. Neuropsychology, with its emphasis on diagnosis, has traditionally had little to offer by way of treatment. In severe brain damage successful methods of cognitive rehabilitation have been developed. But what can neuropsychology offer an individual who is just approaching the threshold of decline?

In response to my patients' prodding to offer them more than a diagnosis, I decided to develop a program to help their cognition. This is not something that I would have embarked on ten years ago. But now, impressed with the evidence reviewed earlier in this book, I felt that the approach was worth a shot.

In designing my program, I followed several principles. First, the program must be diverse, covering a broad range of cognitive functions, including but by no means limited to memory. Executive functions figure prominently in the program. For all the reasons outlined in this book, I felt that executive functions are particularly vulnerable at early stages of cognitive decline. Preserving them to the extent possible is critical for extending cognitive well-being. In addition, I aimed to address as many other cognitive functions as possible.

Second, I decided to stay away from mnemonics and other devices purported to increase the volume of information processing through specialized techniques. Given what we know about the lack of generalization, I felt that there was little to be gained through such approaches. Instead, I wanted the program to offer a cognitive analogue of a gym, to exercise a very broad range of "brain muscles" rather than cognitive skills. The hope has been that engaging the underlying neural machinery will enhance its biological properties. Before enrolling a client into the program, I encouraged him or her to have a neuropsychological evaluation. I tried to tailor the choice of the exercises to the clients' individual patterns of cognitive strengths and weaknesses. Having identified the appropriate cognitive exercises, my colleagues and I assembled them into "comprehensive cognitive workout circuits."

This program is still at an early stage of development—too early to evaluate its efficacy. At the time of this writing, several dozen people have participated in the program, mostly individuals in their sixties and seventies. Virtually without exception, all the participants of this cognitive enhancement program feel that, at a minimum, cognitive exercise gives them an insight into their cognitive strengths and weaknesses. They find this alone empowering and liberating from the fear of dementia. It is equally important that they *like it.* Not a single participant complained that it was a boring chore. In fact, I sometimes joke that I need a forceps to remove some of them from the computer screen when the session is over. So much for computer phobia in the aged!

On the whole, most clients feel that the program confers a genuine cognitive improvement in real-life situations. After vacation breaks they often report a certain loss of cognitive astuteness, which disappears as they rejoin the program. Many of them spread the word, and their friends and acquaintances call and join the program. Frankly, this is more that I expected at the program's inception a few years ago.

Cognitive exercise as a way of preventing mental decline and improving mental functions is uncharted territory. Well, it is almost uncharted. As we move forward along this intriguing new path, we will have to develop both innovative approaches and rigorous methods to evaluate their efficacy. Ideally, one would want to examine the effects of various types of cognitive exercise on brain physiology with the methods of functional neuroimaging. Is there any effect at all? Are the effects global? Are they regional? Are they exercise-dependent? These are important questions, to be addressed by future research in the new century and the new millennium.

12

Frontal Lobes and the Leadership Paradox

Autonomy and Control in the Brain

The frontal lobes are the instrument, and the agent, of control within the central nervous system. It would appear that their advent, late in evolution, should mark a more constrained brain organization. In reality, however, the situation is complex. Several countercurrents unfolded in the evolution of the brain, balancing each other. The evolutionary pressures behind the development of the frontal lobes were probably driven by the increasing degrees of freedom in brain organization and by the impending potential for chaos within it.

Since the early 1980s, the functional organization of the brain has been the focus of intense scientific debate. Two radically different blueprints were being considered. The first blueprint is based on the concept of modularity.[1] As we discussed earlier, a modular system consists of autonomous units, each invested with a relatively complex function and relatively insulated from the others. Separate modules provide inputs to, and receive inputs from, one another, but they exert little or no influence over each other's inner workings. The interaction between modules is limited and gated through a relatively small number of information channels.

The alternative blueprint is a massively parallel, interconnected brain.[2] Here, the units are smaller, invested with far simpler functions, but far more numerous. They are closely interconnected and interact continuously through multiple channels.

The notion of modularity is a high-tech revival of eighteenth-century phrenology. Not only does it presuppose distinct borders between discrete units, but it also suggests their functional prededication. According to this view, a very specific function is rigidly preordained for each such unit.

By contrast, the notion of a massively interconnected brain owes its ascendancy, in a somewhat circular way, to the formal neural networks, or neural nets, which were themselves inspired by the biological nervous system. Neural nets are dynamic models of the brain. They were first introduced in the 1940s, but the advent of computers gave them a recent boost.[3] A neural net is an assembly of a large number of simple interconnected elements, expressed as a computer program. The properties of the elements and connections emulate, in a simplified way, the properties of the real, biological neurons and of the axons and dendrites that interconnect them. By running the program on the computer, the "behavior" of the model challenged with various tasks can be examined, and this allows the examiner to infer the dynamic properties of the real brain. With "experience," the formal neural nets acquire a rich array of properties, which were not explicitly programmed into them from the outset—the "emergent" properties. The patterns of their connection strengths changes, so that various parts of the net form the "representations" of various incoming types of information.

Brain modeling with neural nets is among the most powerful tools of cognitive neuroscience today. The studies of the emergent properties, together with the clinical data about the effects of brain lesions and the methods of functional neuroimaging looking at regional interactions, offer a glimpse into an alternative, amodular principle of brain organization. Earlier in the book, I referred to this principle as gradiental. According to the gradiental principle, massive continuous interactions take place in the brain, while relatively little is preordained about the function of its parts. Instead, it is assumed that the functional roles of various cortical regions *emerge* according to certain basic gradients.[4]

Both the modular and the gradiental concepts have advocates and detractors. Both of them capture important properties of the brain. Modularity is best applicable to an old structure from an evolutionary standpoint, the thalamus, an assemblage of neuronal collections (nuclei). The interactive principle is best applied to a relatively recent evolutionary innovation in the brain, the neocortex. In particular, the interactive principle of organization captures the properties of the most recently evolved part of the neocortex, the so-called heteromodal association cortex, which is critical for the most advanced mental processes. Reptiles and birds are thalamic creatures with little cortical development.[5] This was probably also true for the dinosaurs. Mammals, on the other hand, have a developed cortex, which is superimposed on, and overrides, the thalamus.

The thalamus and the neocortex are closely interconnected. The thalamus is often viewed as the precursor of the cortex, containing in a rudimentary way most of its functions. While functionally close, the thalamus and the neocortex differ radically in neuroanatomical structure. The thalamus consists of distinct nuclei, interconnected with a limited number of pathways as the only routes of communication. By contrast, the neocortex is a sheet without distinct internal borders, with rich pathways interconnecting most areas with most others.

If the thalamus is a close prototype of the cortex, then what were the evolutionary pressures for the emergence of the neocortex? What in evolution promoted the introduction of a fundamentally new principle of neural organization, rather than the refinement of an already existing one? Why was the emergence of a neural sheet, the neocortex, adaptively preferable to sticking with the thalamic principle by having more and larger nuclei? The question is admittedly a teleological one, looking for a "purpose" where there may be none, but we ask teleological questions all the time, putting them in quotation marks so to speak, as intellectual shorthand in our quest for understanding the evolution of complex systems, biological, economic, and social alike.

The probable answer to our teleological question is that different principles of neural organization are optimal for different levels of complexity. Up to a point, modular organization is optimal. But once a certain level of complexity is required, the transition toward a heavily interconnected net consisting of a large number of simpler (but diverse in kind) interactive elements becomes necessary to ensure adaptive success. Throughout evolution, the emphasis has shifted from the brain invested with rigid, fixed functions (the thalamus) to the brain capable of flexible adaptation (the cortex). This was reflected in the explosive neocortical evolution in the mammals.

For sheer combinatorial reasons, the neocortex permits orders-of-magnitude greater numbers of specific connectivity patterns than does a system organized according to the modular principle. Therefore, it is capable of processing a far greater degree of complexity. Furthermore, because the transition from one connectivity pattern to another may occur rapidly in the neocortex, it is characterized by a truly *dynamic topology*.

The transition from the thalamic to the cortical principle of brain organization marks a drastic increase of all possible interaction patterns among different brain structures, neuronal groupings and individual neurons. With this development, the ability to select the most effective pattern in a specific situation becomes particularly important. But the growing degree of freedom available to the brain *in principle* had to be balanced with an effective mechanism of constraining it *at any given time*; otherwise there would be the neural equivalent of chaos.

At the latest stage of cortical evolution the frontal lobes developed to meet this "need." (We remember to put all the teleological allusions in quotation marks.) The type of control provided by the frontal lobes is probably weak, superimposed on a high degree of autonomy of other brain structures. At the same time, the frontal lobe control is "global," coordinating and constraining the activities of a vast array of neural structures at any given time and over time. The frontal lobes do not have the specific knowledge or expertise for all the necessary challenges facing the organism. What they have, however, is the ability to "find" the areas of the brain in possession of this knowledge and expertise for any specific challenge, and to string them together in complex configurations according to the need.

As a neurofuturistic exercise, suppose the evolution of the brain were to continue (in itself a far-from-obvious proposition). Will it continue along the path of increasingly complex and elaborate neural nets, or will a qualitatively new principle of biocomputation emerge? What will it be? An extrapolation based on the foregoing discussion predicts an emergence of a qualitatively more complex and dynamically interconnected network consisting of an order-of-magnitude larger number of smaller components. It is possible, for instance, to envision such a network built of various molecules, rather than neurons, as the basic components.

The principle of man-made molecular biocomputation is already being explored as the basis for the paradigmatic shift in computer design. Life may end up imitating art, the evolution of biological computational systems emulating the evolution of artificial computational devices. But then again it may be precisely the evolution of man-made computational devices that, together with already existing cultural devices of knowledge accumulation and transmission, will make biological evolution of the brain superfluous.

Autonomy and Control in Society

In the spirit of interdisciplinary parallels adopted in this book, I am tempted to apply the analysis of brain evolution to the understanding of the momentous historical changes unfolding before us today. In science the convergence of conclusions based on vastly different sources of knowledge is highly valued. It lends credibility to predictions and points to universal principles underlying diverse complex systems. The search for such universal principles shared by superficially different systems is at the heart of the new field of "complexity" emerging at the cutting edge of science and philosophy. In trying to grasp history, we may be able to draw on the insights of neurobiology. Today a striking parallel is increasingly apparent between the changing world order and the evolution of the brain.

Superficially different yet essentially similar processes are developing in eastern and western Europe. To the east, the Soviet Union has collapsed. Whereas the communist rulers of the fallen Soviet superpower lauded their regime as the dawn of a new era, future historians will view it as the last spasm of the 400-year-old Russian Empire in its middle-of-the-nineteenth-century borders. Farther east, a similar fate may eventually await China.

The Soviet Union disintegrated. Russia has reconstituted itself as an imperial entity incorporating the czarist territorial acquisitions of the sixteenth and seventeenth centuries. Now its constituent ethnic groups are claiming autonomy or even outright independence. This trend took an extreme and particularly destructive form in Chechnya, but the Tatars, Bashkirs, Kalmyks, Yakuts, Ossetians, Dagestans, Ingushis, and others, are also restless. Abkhasians and Mingrels are trying to secede from Georgia. But the fragmentation of the former Soviet Union goes even deeper. During the 1990s, the decade that followed the demise of the Soviet Union, even some of the areas populated mostly by the ethnic Russians began to claim autonomy, and we in the West were hearing about the Kaliningrad Republic, the Urals Republic, and the Maritime Republic of Vladivostok.

Since then, an attempt has been under way to reverse these centrifugal processes and to recentralize the country. It remains to be seen whether these efforts will bring stability and wellbeing to the country or whether, to borrow the bombastic Marxist phrase so familiar to the Russians of my generation, they represent a desperate, and self-defeating, attempt to "turn back the wheel of history" in the name of an imperial ideal whose time has passed. Western political scientists are becoming increasingly aware of the imminent fragmentation of the Russian holdover empire and of the need for new foreign policy approaches in response to it.[6]

In the wake of the collapse of Soviet-controlled or Soviet-inspired regimes, similar changes are unfolding in central Europe. What used to be Czechoslovakia is now Czechia and Slovakia. The fallout of the collapse of Tito's Yugoslavia with its bloody consequences is well known.

In western Europe a resurgence of ethnic factionalism challenges modern nation-states. Provence and Brittany assert their autonomy in France; the Basque country and Catalonia in Spain; Wallonia and Flanders in Belgium; Northern Ireland, Scotland, and Wales in the United Kingdom; northern regions in Italy. As a result, "old tongues are flourishing in a revival of regional cultures."[7] With the blurring of national borders, semiforgotten languages—Breton in Britanny, Gaelic in Scotland, Friulian in northern Italy, Frisian and Limburgs in the Netherlands, Saami in Finland, Basque and Catalan in Spain—are experiencing an unprecedented revival. Increasingly, the claims of cultural revival go beyond a mere quest for cultural autonomy, taking the form of separatism and outright calls for independence.

In both eastern and western Europe, the stable, static, large, and modular nation-states are being replaced by smaller, more fluid political entities. While the events in the east have a clear cause and are perceived in most instances (but with notoriously bloody exceptions) as the process of liberation, the fragmentation in the west is often met with alarm and is more difficult to comprehend. The "medievalization" of Europe is viewed by many as an unwelcome return to a premodern organization.

But could it not be that premodern is also postmodern? One can argue that the phenomena of the East and the West represent the same natural process, and the same dialectic paradox. The paradox is that the demise of strongly integrated nation-states and empires may be the crucial step toward a dynamic, "weakly" integrated Europe and an integrated world. The fragments resulting from this demise are the building blocks of the new order. What seems regressive is really the emergence of a new societal organization, a new spiral in societal evolution. The nature of this transition is elucidated by an analogy with the brain.

If we believe in meaningful parallels between complex systems, then we may use the knowledge of the brain to extrapolate the directions in societal changes, and to a degree the course of history. The transition from the thalamic to the cortical principle of cerebral organization parallels the transition from the macronational to the microregional pattern of societal organization as elements of a global network. In this analogy, the nation-states are modules: autonomous, relatively self-contained entities with interactions regimented and restricted to institutional channels. Today we are witnessing their demise and transition to a new geopolitical order based on a global network comprised of microregional units of organization. The exact nature of future geopolitical entities has yet to reveal itself. Like the components of the brain, they need not be homogeneous and may combine different types of units.

Ethnic regions may become one type of unit of the new order. They are smaller than nation-states and more ancient. Yet their coexistence for the last few centuries within the nation-states and in an increasingly global economy has made them highly interdependent and interactive. A shared history has transformed them from units of isolation into the units of a network. They may become the building blocks of the global politico-economic order transcending national borders. Paradoxically, the shift from the national to ethnic molarity of society may facilitate the shift from a parochial to a global identity, precisely because today ethnicity is less self-sufficient, self-contained, and self-absorbed than nationhood. An ethnic identity may prove easier to reconcile with a pan-European federalist identity than with a national one. As a Basque friend of mine once said, it would be easier for him to forgo his Basque identity in favor of a European identity than in favor of a Spanish one.

Microunits based on strictly economic factors and interrelated through the flows of trade, finance, and communications may emerge as a different type of unit of the evolving new order. This is the conclusion reached by Kenchi Ohmae in *The End of the Nation State.*[8] The proliferation of multinational corporations promotes this type of organization.

The evolution of the brain teaches us the lesson that a high degree of complexity cannot be handled by rigidly organized systems. It requires distributed responsibilities and local autonomy. The arrival of the cortex on the evolutionary scene signaled a true paradigm shift in the organization of the brain. A much more dynamic, faster working central nervous system emerged. This resulted in an exponential surge in the computational power of the brain, which culminated in a conscious mind.

If we follow this analogy, the transition from a world order built of a few large autonomous geopolitical units to a network of many small, highly interdependent geopolitical units is now under way. This transition, too, is nothing short of a paradigm shift. It heralds a new societal dynamism and a quantum leap in the rate of societal change in the centuries to come. This difference is like the difference between a succession of canvases and a kaleidoscope. Far from the end of history proclaimed by some scholars, a much faster moving history is under way.

But in the brain, the advent of the dynamic "new order" ushered in by the advent of the neocortex was balanced by the emergence of the frontal lobes with their ability to superimpose order on an emergent dizzying multitude of possible choices. With an increasing globalization of social and economic interactions, will a similar higher order organization emerge in the global society? What will it be? An improved version of the League of Nations and the United Nations? Some sort of Economic Council of the Multinationals? Is the budding European Union a prototype of such a global organization of "weak" control, with Brussels as the European "prefrontal cortex"? Is a worldwide analogue of the European Union imminent? The brain analogy predicts the eventual emergence of such an organization.

My predictions about the evolution of society based on the brain analogy may sound outlandish and far-fetched. Yet they resonate with some of the cutting-edge thinking of political scientists. My favorite newspaper, the *New York Times,* has again proved to be the best in the world, by providing me with the necessary polemic ammunition. Paul Lewis wrote a review that appeared in the January 2, 1999, issue of the *New York Times* under the provocative title "As Nations Shed Roles,

Is Medieval the Future?"[9] He quotes Hedley Bull, the late professor of international relations at Oxford, predicting that the existing system of nation-states will be replaced by "a modern and secular equivalent of the kind of universal political organization that existed in Western Christendom in the Middle Ages."

The *New York Times* did it again at the very close of the millennium. As my fellow New Yorkers were approaching the year 2000 with the jittery anticipation of millennial frenzy, infrastructure failure, and terrorist attacks, an article titled "Could This Be the New World?" appeared in December 27 issue. In it, Robert Kaplan outlined a doomsday scenario for the century to come: a disintegration of nation-states into a smaller city-states, with the map of the New World becoming a "hologram in constant motion" or, to use the title of his new book, "the coming anarchy."[10] But a mechanism may emerge to offset the coming anarchy through the societal equivalent of the frontal lobes.

A similar argument is made by Stephen J. Kobrin, of the University of Pennsylvania, in a paper in the *Journal of International Affairs*.[11] Kobrin predicts that a "center" of universal authority is bound to emerge to complement the trends toward a growing fragmentation, fluidity, and kaleidoscopic interconnectedness of localities. He points out that most international, intergovernmental organizations were created very recently.

Which form will the postmodern secular analogue of papal authority take? This is a challenge for futurologists to ponder, and the analogy with brain evolution may provide a useful, if not perfectly transparent, "crystal ball."

Autonomy and Control in the Digital World

A peculiar epistemological "man–machine" relationship has developed over the last few decades. It works in both directions. Our insights into the workings of the brain have been informed by the computer analogy during much of the twentieth century, just as they had been by the leading technologies of the time in the centuries past. On the other hand, the design of some of the most powerful computational devices was directly influenced by the brain analogy. The first formal neural nets, designed by McCulloch and Pitts, were directly inspired by the biological neuron analogy; and the design of certain computer languages was directly inspired by the concept of psycholinguistic context.[12]

Consider this intriguing question: Do the biological evolution of the brain and the technological evolution of computers reveal similar guiding principles? If established, such principles will inform us about the ways various, and possibly even most, evolving complex systems cope with increasing computational demands. I will endeavor to show on the next few pages that the transition from a modular principle of organization to a distributed gradiental principle of organization, which seems to characterize the evolution of the brain and society, applies also to the digital world. I will endeavor to show, furthermore, that at a late stage of the evolution of computing, a digital analogue of the frontal lobes has emerged to counterweight the digital "coming anarchy," to borrow Robert Kaplan's anxiety-provoking phrase.[13]

With this demonstration in place, the following intriguing questions arise: Do the invariant laws of evolution shared by the brain, society, and digital computing devices reflect the only intrinsically possible or optimal path of development? Or do humans recapitulate, consciously or unconsciously, their own internal organization in man-made devices and social structures? Each possibility is intriguing in its own right. In the first case, our analysis will point to some very general rules of development of complex systems. In the second case, we encounter a puzzling process of unconscious recapitulation, since neither the evolution of society nor the evolution of the digital world has been explicitly guided by the knowledge of neuroscience.

Computer hardware has evolved from mainframe computers to personal computers to network personal computers. The mainframe computer is a "dinosaur" of the digital world. It occupied several floors of civilian or military research installations. Each mainframe computer had a complex organization and large computational power. It conducted the computation of a task from beginning to end. There were relatively few mainframe computers and the interfaces between them were sparse; they were practically isolated from one another. A digital world dominated by mainframe computers, the 1950s, 1960s, and partly 1970s, was modular in nature. Gradually, however, limited connections between large mainframe computers were created, giving rise to distributed, and ultimately to network, computation.

In the 1970s personal computers (PCs) began to proliferate. The computational power of a single PC is no match to that of a mainframe computer, but there are many more of them. Within this distributed format, a greater range and variety of tasks could be performed. The digital world was no longer dominated by large, functionally prededicated units. It was being taken over by smaller but far more numerous personal computers. To ensure that a maximum number of individual computers could interface, standardization rapidly increased. This signaled the next stage in the evolution of computational devices.

In the 1980s rapid integration of PCs and mainframe computers was taking place. Computational processes were becoming distributed among numerous devices. The multitude of PCs assumed an ever-increasing range of computational tasks, thus reducing, but not totally eliminating, the importance of mainframe computers.

In the 1990s the Internet became ubiquitous. It provided a formal structure for creating interfaces between separate computers according to task demands, within a practically infinite range of combinatorial possibilities. The digital world was becoming increasingly like a neural net. The trend was amplified by the arrival of an entirely different class of computers, "network PCs," limited-capability devices whose main function was to provide access to the Internet. While mainframe computers continued to serve certain functions, a gradual departure from a predominantly modular to a predominantly distributed pattern of organization reshaped the digital world. Both in the evolution of the brain and in the evolution of the digital world a further growth of the computational power of a few self-contained centers proved to be less effective than the development of networks consisting of numerous relatively simple, smaller devices.

But the arrival of "digital anarchy" was not far behind. With the explosion in the volume of information posted on the World Wide Web, finding the specific information required for a particular task became increasingly difficult. As in the evolution of the brain, adaptive pressures arose for the emergence of a mechanism capable of constraining the system's degrees of freedom in any specific, goal-directed situation, while preserving these degrees of freedom in principle. This signaled the invention of "search engines."

Like the frontal lobes, the search engines do not contain the exact knowledge necessary to solve the problem at hand. But like the frontal lobes, they have an aerial view of the system, which enables them to find the specific locations within the net where this knowledge is held. And like the frontal lobes, the search engines appeared at a relatively late stage of transition of the digital world from a mostly modular to a mostly distributed "organism." Search engines provide the executive function within the Internet. They are the *digital frontal lobes.*

So it appears that strong similarities exist between the evolution of the brain, society, and man-made computational systems. Each is characterized by a transition from the modular principle of organization to the distributed, gradiental principle. At a highly evolved stage of this process, a system of "executive" control emerges, to help rein in the prospect of anarchy and chaos, which paradoxically increases with the increase of any system's complexity. The peculiar relationship between autonomy and control embodied in the executive control exerted by the frontal lobes was captured in the quotable phrase coined by Frederick Engels: "Freedom is necessity recognized."[14]

Epilogue

At the time I wrote this book I had lived almost precisely equal parts of my life in the East and in the West, and by most realistic projections I had entered its final third—the time of integration, an executive task indeed. In retrospect, my own intellectual journey has been an amalgam and a melding of influences derived from these two worlds, and to the extent that I can claim an intellectual and scientific style of my own, it was shaped by this fusion. I am a man of the East in the Western cultural cloth, so to speak. At the beginning of my life's sixth decade a nomad in me reasserted himself. I run my clinical practice in New York, do my research in Sydney, and lecture worldwide.

And for the first time since I left Russia a quarter of a century ago, I find myself feeling a keen interest in its flawed stumble toward a more enlightened paradigm of economy and governance. I am aided in the writing of this book, in my research, and in my clinical practice by my three Russian assistants, Dmitri, Peter, and Sergey, operating out of my mid-Manhattan office, all young people representing that culture's future and not its past. The lives of the close friends in whom many years ago I had confided my plans to leave the place have diverged professionally and personally, reflecting the changes that transformed Russia since I left it. Peter Tulviste became the first postindependence president of Tartu University in his native, finally free, Estonia. Slavik Danilov is a colonel and professor of psychology at a uniformed services academy in Russia. Natasha Korsakova is a leading researcher of Alzheimer's dementia and teaches at Moscow State University. Lena Moskovich lives in Boston, where she conducts research in behavioral neurology. Ekhtibar Dzafarov also left Russia and has taught at various universities in Europe and in the United States.

And when this book is finally written, I plan a trip to Moscow, the first since I left it when it was the capital of a different country. I will take a walk down the streets where I had my fateful conversation with Alexandr Romanovich, and some of the streets will have different names, the Soviet pantheon having been cast away; but others, like Arbat, will remain. I will visit friends and try to reconnect to the place of my youth and to get a sense of the new Russia. Then I will return home to New York, but hopefully with the feeling that what used to be my home is no longer a strange place.

This book began with the discussion of the brain and ended with the discussion of society and history. The paradigm has been reversed. It is common in the history of ideas to use the concepts of a more mature science as a heuristic metaphor for a more embryonic one. For centuries neuroscience has been the embryonic science borrowing its metaphors from more evolved disciplines: from mechanics (hydraulic pumps of the seventeenth century), electric engineering (the telephone switchboard of the early twentieth century), and computer science (the second half of the twentieth century). But now brain science is coming of age and it may be ready to offer its own heuristic metaphors to shed light on other complex systems, including society.

Brain science has always been on the border of hard science and the humanities, and it is precisely this fusion that drew me to it many years ago. The name of Descartes is often mentioned when the history of brain–mind exploration is examined. But I drew my early inspiration from Descartes's contemporary, and a fellow iconoclast, Baruch Spinoza.[1] Unlike Descartes, Spinoza did not believe in the duality of spirit and matter. He understood God as the fundamental laws of the universe and not as its creator, and he searched for unifying principles.

At the age of 12, browsing through my father's library, as I often did, I stumbled onto a two-volume Russian translation of Spinoza's *Ethics,* the first time I heard of the man. As I was poring through the obscure writings, I came upon his "ethics theorems proved with deductive method."[2] As my personal cognitive history goes, this was one of its most powerful moments. I had always been drawn to mathematics and to the humanities and history, but not particularly to natural sciences—an uncommon configuration of interests. And I was clearly interested in the life of the mind, but famously unimpressed with what little I knew at the time of psychology as a discipline. Spinoza was a revelation to me, telling me that these disparate areas could be brought together and that the seemingly inherently imprecise subjects like the mind, society, and the life of the mind in society could be approached with precise methods.

Of course, Spinoza's seventeenth-century enterprise was naive by today's standards. Nor did it exert, to my knowledge, a major influence on shaping the studies of complex systems like the brain or society into the relatively precise disciplines that they have become. Many more direct and influential efforts of the kind existed, of which I was not aware at the time. But to me that early encounter with Spinoza was a formative experience, which more than any single influence encouraged my choice of psychology and neuroscience as a lifelong career.

Another intellectual encounter of comparable potency occurred much later, when at the age of 19 I stumbled at the Moscow State University library into the classic papers by Warren McCulloch and Walter Pitts titled "A Logical Calculus of the Ideas Immanent in Nervous Activity" (1943)[3] and "How We Know Universals: The Perception of Auditory and Visual Forms"(1947),[4] laying the groundwork for formal neural net modeling of the brain. To me, there was a clear intellectual continuity between Spinoza's "ethics theorems" and McCulloch and Pitts's "logical calculus." Each represented an attempt to infuse traditionally vague inquiry into the mind and the brain with precise deductive method. Very little was happening at the time in Russia of what was later to be called "computational neuroscience." With Luria's amused acquiescence, my friend Yelena Artemyeva, a brilliant mathematician and a student of Andrey Kolmogorov, and I tried to introduce neural net modeling into the neuropsychological research at University of Moscow.

My subsequent life in the United States took me much further away from basic research and toward clinical work than I had anticipated in those early years of my career. But my understanding of the brain, and the heuristic metaphor that guided that understanding, has always been informed by the early intellectual encounter with the concept of the neural net.

Following these early influences and throughout my career I

have been interested, sometimes explicitly and sometimes tacitly, in general principles that transcend my own relatively narrow field of knowledge. And so it seems an intellectual full circle of sorts: my own idiosyncratic understanding of the brain produced a metaphor that was useful to me personally in understanding the cataclysmic societal phenomena through which we live. I hope that the metaphor will be useful to other people.

I believe that the discussion of the relationship between autonomy and control in various complex systems and the lessons drawn from the analysis of the brain for the understanding of society is a fitting way to end this book. No complex system can succeed without an effective executive mechanism, the "frontal lobes." But the frontal lobes operate best as part of a highly distributed, interactive structure with much autonomy and many degrees of freedom.

References and Notes

Chapter 1: Introduction

1. A. Damasio, *Descartes' Error: Emotion, Reason, and the Human Brain* (New York: Putnam Publishing Group, 1994).

2. R. A. Barkley, *ADHD and the Nature of Self-Control* (New York: Guilford Press, 1997).

3. E. Goldberg, "Tribute to Alexandr Romanovich Luria," in *Contemporary Neuropsychology and the Legacy of Luria*, ed. E. Goldberg (Hillsdale, New Jersey: Lawrence Erlbaum Associates, 1990), 1–9.

4. S. Sontag, *Illness as Metaphor and AIDS and Its Metaphors* (New York: Doubleday Books, 1990).

Chapter 2: An End and a Beginning: A Dedication

1. Following the demise of the Soviet Union, streets and public places named after the Soviet demigods and memorable dates have been changed, in most instances given their prerevolutionary names.

Chapter 3: The Brain's Chief Executive: The Frontal Lobes at a Glance

1. For the transformation of military leadership through history, see J. Keegan, *The Mask of Command* (New York: Penguin, 1989).

2. Napoleon's chronic illness had no direct relationship to his brain. Quite the opposite, it entailed greatly inflamed hemorrhoids. For further reading, see

A. Neumayr, *Dictators in the Mirror of Medicine: Napoleon, Hitler, Stalin,* trans. D. J. Parent (Bloomington, Illinois: Medi-Ed Press, 1995).

3. F. Tilney, *The Brain: From Ape to Man* (New York: Hoeber, 1928).

4. J. Jaynes, *The Origin of Consciousness in the Breakdown of the Bicameral Mind* (New York: Houghton Mifflin Company, 1990).

5. Quoted in W. E. Wallace, Michelangelo: *The Complete Sculpture, Painting, Architecture* (Southport, Connecticut: Hugh Lauter Levin Associates, 1998).

6. S. Pinker, *The Language Instinct* (New York: Harper Perennial Library, 1995).

Chapter 4: Architecture of the Brain: A Primer

1. For more thorough review see A. Parent, *Carpenter's Human Neuroanatomy,* 9th ed. (Baltimore: Williams & Wilkins, 1995). (Revised edition of M. B. Carpenter and J. Satin, *Human Neuroanatomy,* 8th ed, 1983.)

2. H. W. Magoun, "The ascending reticular activating system," *Res Publ Assoc Nerv Ment Dis,* no. 30 (1952).

3. Thorough review on this topic can be found in D. Oakley and H. Plotkin, eds., *Brain, Behavior and Evolution* (Cambridge, UK: Cambridge University Press, 1979).

4. Again, for more thorough review see A. Parent, *Carpenter's Human Neuroanatomy,* 9th ed. (Baltimore: Williams & Wilkins, 1995).

5. Ibid.

6. J. LeDoux, *The Emotional Brain: The Mysterious Underpinnings of Emotional Life* (New York: Touchstone Books, 1998).

7. J. Grafman, I. Litvan, S. Massaquoi, M. Stewart, A. Sirigu, M. Hallett, "Cognitive planning deficit in patients with cerebellar atrophy," *Neurology* 42, no. 8 (1992): 1493–1496; H. C. Leiner, A. L. Leiner, and R. S. Dow, "Reappraising the cerebellum: what does the hindbrain contribute to the forebrain?" *Behav Neurosci* 103, no. 5 (1989): 998–1008.

8. In D. Oakley and H. Plotkin, eds., *Brain, Behavior and Evolution* (Cambridge, UK: Cambridge University Press, 1979).

9. B. L. McNaughton and R. G. M Morris, "Hippocampal synaptic enhancement and information storage," *Trends Neurosci* 10 (1987): 408–415; B. L. McNaughton, "Associative pattern competition in hippocampal circuits: new evidence and new questions," *Brain Res Rev* 16 (1991): 202–204.

10. B. Milner, "Cues to the cerebral organization of memory," in *Cerebral Correlates of Conscious Experience,* ed. P. Buser and A. Rougeul-Buser (Amsterdam: Elsevier, 1978), 139–153.

11. In C. H. Hockman, ed., *Limbic System Mechanisms and Autonomic Function* (Springfield, Illinois: Charles C Thomas, 1972).

12. C. S. Carter, M. M. Botvinick, and J. D. Cohen, "The contribution of the anterior cingulate cortex to executive processes in cognition," *Rev Neurosci* 10, no. 1 (1999): 49–57.

13. In D. Oakley and H. Plotkin, eds., *Brain, Behavior and Evolution* (Cambridge, UK: Cambridge University Press, 1979).

14. K. Brodmann, *Vergleichende Lokalisationslehre der Grosshinrinde in ihren*

Prinzipien dargestellt auf Grund des Zellenbaues (Leipzig: Barth, 1909). Cited in J. M. Fuster, *The Prefrontal Cortex: Anatomy, Physiology, and Neuropsychology of the Frontal Lobe,* 3rd ed. (Philadelphia: Lippincott–Raven, 1997).

15. G. W. Roberts, P. N. Leigh, D. R. Weinberger, *Neuropsychiatric Disorders* (London: Wolfe, 1993).

16. J. M. Fuster, *The Prefrontal Cortex: Anatomy, Physiology, and Neuropsychology of the Frontal Lobe,* 3rd ed. (Philadelphia: Lippincott–Raven, 1997).

17. In A. W. Campbell, *Histological Studies on the Localization of Cerebral Function* (Cambridge: Cambridge University Press, 1905). Cited in J. M. Fuster, *The Prefrontal Cortex: Anatomy, Physiology, and Neuropsychology of the Frontal Lobe,* 3rd ed. (Philadelphia: Lippincott–Raven, 1997).

18. J. H. Jackson, "Evolution and dissolution of the nervous system," *Croonian Lecture. Selected Papers* 2 (1884).

19. A. R. Luria, *Higher Cortical Functions in Man* (New York: Basic Books, 1966).

20. A. Damasio, "The frontal lobes," in *Clinical Neuropsychology,* ed. K. Heilman and E. Valenstein (New York: Oxford University Press, 1993), 360–412.

21. J. M. Fuster, *The Prefrontal Cortex: Anatomy, Physiology, and Neuropsychology of the Frontal Lobe,* 3rd ed. (Philadelphia: Lippincott–Raven, 1997).

22. P. S. Goldman-Rakic, "Circuitry of primate prefrontal cortex and regulation of behavior by representational memory," in *Handbook of Physiology: Nervous System, Higher Functions of the Brain,* Part 1, ed. F. Plum (Bethesda, Maryland: American Physiological Association, 1987), 373–417.

23. D. T. Stuss and D. F. Benson, *The Frontal Lobes* (New York: Raven Press, 1986).

24. W. J. Nauta, "Neural associations of the frontal cortex," *Acta Neurobiol Exp* 32, no. 2 (1972): 125–140.

25. J. H. Jackson, "Evolution and dissolution of the nervous system," *Croonian Lecture. Selected Papers* 2 (1884).

Chapter 5: The Orchestra's Front Row: The Cortex

1. F. J. Gall, *Sur le fonctions du cerveau,* 6 vols. (Paris, 1822–1823).

2. K. Kleist, *Gehirnpathologie* (Leipzig: Barth, 1934).

3. P. Broca, "Remarques sur le siège de la faculté du language articule," *Bull Soc Anthrop* 6 (1861).

4. C. Wernicke, *Der aphasische Symptomencomplex* (Breslau, 1874).

5. M. LeMay, "Morphological cerebral asymmetries of modern man, fossil man, and nonhuman primate," *Ann N Y Acad Sci* 280 (1976): 349–366.

6. M. C. de Lacoste, D. S. Horvath, and D. J. Woodward, "Possible sex differences in the developing human fetal brain," *J Clin Exp Neuropsychol* 13, no. 6 (1991): 831–846.

7. M. LeMay, "Morphological cerebral asymmetries of modern man, fossil man, and nonhuman primate," *Ann N Y Acad Sci* 280 (1976): 349–366.

8. M. C. Diamond, "Rat forebrain morphology: right–left; male–female; young–old; enriched–impoverished," in *Cerebral Laterality in Nonhuman Species,* ed. S. D. Glick (New York: Academic Press, 1985); M. C. Diamond, G. A. Dowl-

ing, and R. E. Johnson, "Morphologic cerebral cortical asymmetry in male and female rats," *Exp Neurol* 71, no. 2 (1981): 261–268.

9. N. Geschwind and W. Levitsky, "Human brain: left–right asymmetries in temporal speech region," *Science* 161, no. 837 (1968): 186–187.

10. M. LeMay and N. Geschwind, "Hemispheric differences in the brains of great apes," *Brain Behav Evol* 11, no. 1 (1975): 48–52.

11. P. J. Gannon et al., "Asymmetry of chimpanzee planum temporale: humanlike pattern of Wernicke's brain language area homolog," *Science* 279, no. 5348 (1998): 220–222.

12. S. D. Glick, D. A. Ross, and L. B. Hough, "Lateral asymmetry of neurotransmitters in human brain," *Brain Res* 234, no. 1 (1982): 53–63.

13. S. Sandu, P. Cook, and M. C. Diamond, "Rat cortical estrogen receptors: male–female, right–left," Exp Neurol 92, no. 1 (1985): 186–196.

14. S. D. Glick, R. C. Meibach, R. D. Cox, S. Maayani, "Multiple and interrelated functional asymmetries in rat brain," *Life Sci* 25, no. 4 (1979): 395–400.

15. S. A. Sholl and K. L. Kim, "Androgen receptors are differentially distributed between right and left cerebral hemispheres of the fetal male rhesus monkey," *Brain Res* 516, no. 1 (1990): 122–126.

16. E. Goldberg and L. D. Costa, "Hemisphere differences in the acquisition and use of descriptive systems," *Brain Lang* 14, no. 1 (1981): 144–173.

17. H. Simon, *The Sciences of the Artificial* (Cambridge: MIT Press, 1996).

18. S. Grossberg, ed., *Neural Networks and Natural Intelligence* (Cambridge: MIT Press, 1988).

19. E. Goldberg and L. D. Costa, "Hemisphere differences in the acquisition and use of descriptive systems," *Brain Lang* 14, no. 1 (1981): 144–173.

20. For relevant computational models utilizing formal neural nets see S. Grossberg, ed., *Neural Networks and Natural Intelligence* (Cambridge: MIT Press, 1988); R. A. Jacobs and M. I. Jordan, "Computational consequences of a bias toward short connections," *J Cogn Neurosc* 4 (1992): 323–336; R. A. Jacobs, M. I. Jordan, and A. G. Barto, "Task decomposition through competition in a modular connectionist architecture: the what and where vision tasks," *Cognit Sci* 15 (1991): 219–250.

21. For review see S. Springer and G. Deutsch, *Left Brain, Right Brain: Perspective from Cognitive Neuroscience*, 5th ed. (New York: W H Freeman & Co, 1997).

22. T. G. Bever and R. J. Chiarello, "Cerebral dominance in musicians and nonmusicians," *Science* 185, no. 150 (1974): 537–539.

23. C. A. Marzi and G. Berlucchi, "Right visual field superiority for accuracy of recognition of famous faces in normals," *Neuropsychologia* 15, no. 6 (1977): 751–756.

24. A. Martin, C. L. Wiggs, and J. Weisberg, "Modulation of human medial temporal lobe activity by form, meaning, and experience," *Hippocampus* 7, no. 6 (1997): 587–593.

25. R. Henson, T. Shallice, and R. Dolan, "Neuroimaging evidence for dissociable forms of repetition priming," *Science* 287, no. 5456 (2000): 1269–1272.

26. J. M. Gold et al., "PET validation of a novel prefrontal task: delayed response alteration," *Neuropsychology* 10 (1996): 3–10.

27. R. Shadmehr and H. H. Holcomb, "Neural correlates of motor memory consolidation," *Science* 277, no. 5327 (1997): 821–825.

28. R. J. Haier, B. V., Siegel Jr., A. MacLachlan, E. Soderling, S. Lottenberg, M. S. Buchsbaum, "Regional glucose metabolic changes after learning a complex visuospatial/motor task: a positron emission tomographic study," *Brain Res* 570, no. 1–2 (1992): 134–143.

29. G. S. Berns, J. D. Cohen, and M. A. Mintun, "Brain regions responsive to novelty in the absence of awareness," *Science* 276, no. 5316 (1997): 1272–1275.

30. M. E. Raichle, J. A. Fiez, T. O. Videen, A. M. MacLeod, J. V. Pardo, P. T. Fox, S. E. Petersen, "Practice-related changes in human brain functional anatomy during nonmotor learning," *Cereb Cortex* 4, no. 1 (1994): 26.

31. E. Tulving, H. J. Markowitsch, F. E. Craik, R. Hiabib, S. Houle, "Novelty and familiarity activations in PET studies of memory encoding and retrieval," *Cereb Cortex* 6, no. 1 (1996): 71–79.

32. L. Vygotsky, *Thought and Language*, ed. A. Kozulin (Cambridge: MIT Press, 1986).

33. J. Jaynes, *The Origin of Consciousness in the Breakdown of the Bicameral Mind* (New York: Houghton Mifflin Company, 1990).

34. J.M. Gold, K. F. Berman, C. Randolph, T. E. Goldberg, D. Weinberger, "PET validation of a novel prefrontal task: delayed response alteration," *Neuropsychology* 10 (1996): 3–10; R. J. Haier et al., "Regional glucose metabolic changes after learning a complex visuospatial/motor task: a positron emission tomographic study," *Brain Res* 570, no. 1–2 (1992): 134–143; M. E. Raichle, J. A. Fiez, T. O. Videen, A. M. MacLeod, J. V. Pardo, P. T. Fox, S. E. Petersen, "Practice-related changes in human brain functional anatomy during nonmotor learning," *Cereb Cortex* 4, no. 1 (1994): 8–26.

35. J. A. Fodor, "Precis of the modularity of mind," *Behav Brain Sci* 8 (1985): 1–42.

36. E. Goldberg, "Gradiental approach to neocortical functional organization," *J Clin Exp Neuropsychol* 11, no. 4 (1989): 489–517.

37. E. Goldberg, "Higher cortical functions in humans: the gradiental approach," in *Contemporary Neuropsychology and the Legacy of Luria*, ed. E. Goldberg (Hillsdale, New Jersey: Lawrence Erlbaum Associates, 1990), 229–276.

38. O. W. Sacks, "Scotoma: forgetting and neglect in science," in *Hidden Histories of Science*, ed. R. B. Silver (New York: New York Review, 1996), 141–187.

39. For review see K. Heilman and E. Valenstein, eds., *Clinical Neuropsychology* (New York: Oxford University Press, 1993).

40. E. Goldberg, "Associative agnosias and the functions of the left hemisphere," *J Clin Exp Neuropsychol* 12, no. 4 (1990): 467–484.

41. E. Goldberg, "Gradiental approach to neocortical functional organization," *J Clin Exp Neuropsychol* 11, no. 4 (1989): 489–517.

42. A. Martin, L. G. Ungerleider, and J. V. Haxby, "Category specificity and the brain: the sensory/motor model of semantic representation of objects," in *The New Cognitive Neuroscience*, ed. M. S. Gazzaniga (Cambridge: MIT Press, 1999).

43. A. Martin, C. L. Wiggs, L. G. Ungerleider, J. V. Haxby, "Neural correlates of category-specific knowledge," *Nature* 379, no. 6566 (1996): 649–652.

44. E. K. Warrington and T. Shallice, "Category specific semantic impairments," *Brain* 107, no. 3 (1984): 829–854; R. A. McCarthy and E. K. Warrington, "Evidence for modality-specific meaning systems in the brain," *Nature* 334, no. 6181 (1988): 428–30.

Chapter 6: The Conductor: A Closer Look at the Frontal Lobes

1. M. E. Raichle, J. A. Fiez, T. O. Videen, A. M. MacLeod, J. V. Pardo, P. T. Fox, S. E. Petersen, "Practice-related changes in human brain functional anatomy during nonmotor learning," *Cereb Cortex* 4, no. 1 (1994): 8–26.

2. J. M. Gold, K. F. Berman, C. Randolph, T. E. Goldberg, D. Weinberger, "PET validation of a novel prefrontal task: delayed response alteration," *Neuropsychology* 10 (1996): 3–10.

3. C. F. Jacobsen, "Functions of the frontal association area in primates," *Arch Neurol Psychiatry* 33 (1935): 558–569; C. F. Jacobsen and H. W. Nissen, "Studies of cerebral function in primates: IV. The effects of frontal lobe lesion on the delayed alternation habit in monkeys," *J Comp Physiol Psychol* 23 (1937): 101–112.

4. A. R. Luria, *Higher Cortical Functions in Man* (New York: Basic Books, 1966).

5. P. S. Goldman-Rakic, "Circuitry of primate prefrontal cortex and regulation of behavior by representational memory," in *Handbook of Physiology: Nervous System, Higher Functions of the Brain,* Part 1, ed. F. Plum (Bethesda, Maryland: American Physiological Association, 1987), 373–417.

6. J. M. Fuster, *The Prefrontal Cortex: Anatomy, Physiology, and Neuropsychology of the Frontal Lobe,* 3rd ed. (Philadelphia: Lippincott–Raven, 1997).

7. J. M. Fuster, "Temporal organization of behavior (Introduction)," *Hum Neurobiol* 4 (1985): 57–60.

8. J. H. Jackson, "Evolution and dissolution of the nervous system," *Croonian Lecture. Selected Papers* 2 (1884).

9. S. Funahashi, C. J. Bruce, and P. S. Goldman-Rakic, "Mnemonic coding of visual space in the monkey's dorsolateral prefrontal cortex," *J Neurophysiol* 61, no. 2 (1989): 331–349.

10. S. M. Courtney, L. G. Ungerleider, K. Keil, J. V. Haxby, "Object and spatial visual working memory activate separate neural systems in human cortex," *Cereb Cortex* 6, no. 1 (1996): 39–49.

11. S. Funahashi, C. J. Bruce, and P. S. Goldman-Rakic, "Mnemonic coding of visual space in the monkey's dorsolateral prefrontal cortex," *J Neurophysiol* 61, no. 2 (1989): 331–349.

12. E. Goldberg, R. Harner, M. Lovell, K. Podell, S. Riggio, "Cognitive bias, functional cortical geometry, and the frontal lobes: laterality, sex, and handedness," *J Cogn Neurosci* 6, no. 3 (1994): 276–296.

13. E. Goldberg, A. Kluger, T. Griesing, L. Malta, M. Shapiro, S. Ferris, "Early diagnosis of frontal-lobe dementias." Presented at the Eighth Congress of the International Psychogeriatric Association; August 17–22, Jerusalem, Israel.

14. For review see B. Reisberg, ed., *Alzheimer's Disease* (New York: The Free Press, 1983).

Chapter 7: Different Lobes for Different Folks: Decision-Making Styles and the Frontal Lobes

1. J. Talairach and P. Tournoux, *Co-planar Stereotaxic Atlas of the Human Brain* (New York: Thieme, 1988).

2. R. P. Ebstein, O. Novick, R. Umansky, B. Priel, Y. Osher, D. Blaine, E. R. Bennett, L. Nemanov, M. Katz, R. H. Belmaker, "Dopamine D4 receptor (D4DR) exon III polymorphism associated with the human personality trait of novelty seeking," *Nat Genet* 12, no. 1 (1996): 78–80.

3. E. Goldberg, R. Harner, M. Lovell, K. Podell, S. Riggio, "Cognitive bias, functional cortical geometry, and the frontal lobes: laterality, sex, and handedness," *J Cogn Neurosci* 6, no. 3 (1994): 276–296.

4. M. LeMay, "Morphological cerebral asymmetries of modern man, fossil man, and nonhuman primate," *Ann N Y Acad Sci* 280 (1976): 349–366.

5. M. C. Diamond, "Rat forebrain morphology: right–left; male–female; young–old; enriched–impoverished," in *Cerebral Laterality in Nonhuman Species*, ed. S. D. Glick (New York: Academic Press, 1985); M. C. Diamond, G. A. Dowling, and R. E. Johnson, "Morphologic cerebral cortical asymmetry in male and female rats," *Exp Neurol* 71, no. 2 (1981): 261–268; S. D. Glick, R. C. Meibach, R. D. Cox, S. Maayani, "Multiple and interrelated functional asymmetries in rat brain," *Life Sci* 25, no. 4 (1979): 395–400; S. D. Glick, D. A. Ross, and L. B. Hough, "Lateral asymmetry of neurotransmitters in human brain," *Brain Res* 234, no. 1 (1982): 53–63.

6. S. D. Glick, D. A. Ross, and L. B. Hough, "Lateral asymmetry of neurotransmitters in human brain," *Brain Res* 234, no. 1 (1982): 53–63; S. Sandu, P. Cook, and M. C. Diamond, "Rat cortical estrogen receptors: male–female, right–left," *Exp Neurol* 92, no. 1 (1985): 186–196.

7. S. D. Glick, D. A. Ross, and L. B. Hough, "Lateral asymmetry of neurotransmitters in human brain," *Brain Res* 234, no. 1 (1982): 53–63.

8. For review see E. Goldberg, R. Harner, M. Lovell, K. Podell, S. Riggio, "Cognitive bias, functional cortical geometry, and the frontal lobes: laterality, sex, and handedness," *J Cogn Neurosci* 6, no. 3 (1994): 276–296; S. Springer and G. Deutsch, *Left Brain, Right Brain: Perspective from Cognitive Neuroscience*, 5th ed. (New York: W H Freeman & Co, 1997); D. W. Lewis and M. C. Diamond, "The influence of the gonadal steroids on the assymetry of the cerebral cortex," in *Brain Assymetry*, ed. R. J. Davidson and K. Hugdahl (Cambridge: MIT Press, 1995), 31–50.

9. K. S. Kendler and D. Walsh, "Gender and schizophrenia: results of an epidemiologically-based family study," *Br J Psychiatry* 167, no. 2 (1995): 184–192.

10. E. Shapiro, A. K. Shapiro, and J. Clarkin, "Clinical psychological testing in Tourette's syndrome," *J Pers Assess* 38, no. 5 (1974): 464–478.

11. S. L. Andersen and M. H. Teicher, "Sex differences in dopamine receptors and their relevance to ADHD," *Neurosci Biobehav Rev* 24, no. 1 (2000): 137–141.

12. S. K. Min, S. K. An, D. I. Jon, J. D. Lee, "Positive and negative symptoms and regional cerebral perfusion in antipsychotic-naive schizophrenic patients: a high-resolution SPECT study," *Psychiatry Res* 90, no. 3 (1999): 159–168; R. E. Gur, S. M. Resnick, and R. C. Gur, "Laterality and frontality of cerebral blood flow and metabolism in schizophrenia: relationship to symptom specificity," *Psychiatry Res* 27, no. 3 (1989): 325–334.

13. P. Flor-Henry, "The obsessive-compulsive syndrome: reflection of fronto-caudate dysregulation of the left hemisphere?" *Encephale* 16 (special issue) (1990): 325–329.

14. L. Baving, M. Laucht, and M. H. Schmidt, "Atypical frontal brain acti-

vation in ADHD: preschool and elementary school boys and girls," *J Am Acad Child Adolesc Psychiatry* 38, no. 11 (1999): 1363–1371.

15. E. Goldberg, R. Harner, M. Lovell, K. Podell, S. Riggio, "Cognitive bias, functional cortical geometry, and the frontal lobes: laterality, sex, and handedness," *J Cogni Neurosc* 6, no. 3 (1994): 276–296.

16. D. Kimura, "Sex differences in cerebral organization for speech and praxic functions," *Can J Psychol* 37, no. 1 (1983): 19–35.

17. F. B. Wood, D. L. Flowers, and C. E. Naylor, "Cerebral laterality in functional neuroimaging," in *Cerebral Laterality: Theory and Research. The Toledo Symposium,* ed. F. L. Kittle (Hillsdale, New Jersey: Lawrence Erlbaum Associates, 1991), 103–115.

18. B. A. Shaywitz, S. E. Shaywitz, K. R. Pugh, R. T. Constable, P. Skudlarski, R. K. Fulbright, R. A. Bronen, J. M. Fletcher, D. P. Shankweiler, L. Katz, "Sex differences in the functional organization of the brain for language," *Nature* 373, no. 6515 (1995): 607–609.

19. S. F. Witelson, "The brain connection: the corpus callosum is larger in left-handers," *Science* 229 (1985): 665–668; M. Habib, D. Gayraud, A. Oliva, J. Regis, G. Salamon, R. Khalil, "Effects of handedness and sex on the morphology of the corpus callosum: a study with brain magnetic resonance imaging," *Brain Cogn* 16, no. 1 (1991): 41–61.

20. J. Harasty, K. L. Double, G. M. Halliday, J. J. Krill, D. A. McRitchie, "Language-associated cortical regions are proportionally larger in the female brain," *Arch Neurol* 54, no. 2 (1997): 171–176; J. Harasty, "Language processing in both sexes: evidence from brain studies," *Brain* 123, no. 2 (2000): 404–406.

21. M. Mishkin and K. H. Pribram, "Analysis of the effects of frontal lesions in monkeys: I. Variations of delayed alterations," *J Comp Physiol Psychol* 48 (1955): 492–495; M. Mishkin and K. H. Pribram, "Analysis of the effects of frontal lesions in the monkey: II. Variations of delayed response," *J Comp Physiol Psychol* 49 (1956): 36–40.

22. E. Goldberg, R. Harner, M. Lovell, K. Podell, S. Riggio, "Cognitive bias, functional cortical geometry, and the frontal lobes: laterality, sex, and handedness," *J Cogn Neurosci* 6, no. 3 (1994): 276–296.

23. J. Bradshaw and L. Rogers, *The Evolution of Lateral Assymetries, Language, Tool Use, and Intellect* (San Diego: Academic Press, 1993).

24. S. Springer and G. Deutsch, *Left Brain, Right Brain: Perspective from Cognitive Neuroscience,* 5th ed. (New York: W H Freeman & Co, 1997).

25. Ibid.

26. Personal communication from Mortimer Mishkin. 1994.

27. E. Goldberg, R. Harner, M. Lovell, K. Podell, S. Riggio, "Cognitive bias, functional cortical geometry, and the frontal lobes: laterality, sex, and handedness," *J Cogn Neurosci* 6, no. 3 (1994): 276–296.

28. R. P. Ebstein, O. Novik, R. Umansky, B. Priez, Y. Osher, D. Blaine, E. R. Bennett, L. Nemanov, M. Katz, R. M. Bellmaker, "Dopamine D4 receptor (D4DR) exon III polymorphism associated with the human personality trait of novelty seeking," *Nat Genet* 12, no. 1 (1996): 78–80; J. Benjamin et al., "Population and familial association between the D4 dopamine receptor gene and measures of novelty seeking," *Nat Genet* 12, no. 1 (1996): 81–84.

29. D. L. Orsini and P. Satz, "A syndrome of pathological left-handedness: correlates of early left hemisphere injury," *Arch Neurol* 43, no. 4 (1986): 333–337;

P. Satz, P. Cook, M. C. Diamond, "The pathological left-handedness syndrome," *Brain Cogn* 4, no. 1 (1985): 27–46.

30. G. Rajkowska and P. S. Goldman-Rakic, "Cytoarchitectonic definition of prefrontal areas in the normal human cortex: II. Variability in locations of areas 9 and 46 and relationship to the Talairach Coordinate System," *Cereb Cortex* 5, no. 4 (1995): 323–337; G. Rajkowska and P. S. Goldman-Rakic, "Cytoarchitectonic definition of prefrontal areas in the normal human cortex: I. Remapping of areas 9 and 46 using quantitative criteria," *Cereb Cortex* 5, no. 4 (1995): 307–322.

31. H. E. Gardner, *Multiple Intelligences: The Theory in Practice* (New York: Basic Books, 1993).

32. D. Goleman, *Emotional Intelligence* (New York: Bantam Books, 1997).

33. S. J. Gould, *The Mismeasure of Man* (New York: W W Norton, 1981).

34. S. F. Witelson, D. L. Kigar, and T. Harvey, "The exceptional brain of Albert Einstein," *Lancet* 353, no. 9170 (1999): 2149–2153.

35. C. D. Frith and U. Frith, "Interacting minds: a biological basis," *Science* 286, no. 5445 (1999): 1692–1695.

36. Ibid.

37. G. G. Gallup Jr., "Absence of self-recognition in a monkey (*Macaca fascicularis*) following prolonged exposure to a mirror," *Dev Psychobiol* 10, no. 3 (1977): 281–284; M. D. Hauser, J. Kralik, C. Botto-Mahan, M. Garrett, J. Oser, "Self-recognition in primates: phylogeny and the salience of species-typical features," *Proc Natl Acad Sci U S A* 92, no. 23 (1995): 10811–10814.

38. M. D. Hauser et al., "Self-recognition in primates: phylogeny and the salience of species-typical features," *Proc Natl Acad Sci U S A* 92, no. 23 (1995): 10811–10814.

39. C. D. Frith and U. Frith, "Interacting minds: a biological basis," Science 286, no. 5445 (1999): 1692–1695.

40. J. Jaynes, *The Origin of Consciousness in the Breakdown of the Bicameral Mind* (New York: Houghton Mifflin Company, 1990).

41. Ibid.

Chapter 8: When the Leader Is Wounded

1. A. Damasio, *Descartes' Error; Emotion, Reason, and the Human Brain* (New York: Putnam Publishing Group, 1994).

2. E. Goldberg, "Introduction: the frontal lobes in neurological and psychiatric conditions," *Neuropsychiatry Neuropsychol Behav Neurol* 5, no. 4 (1992): 231–232.

3. Ibid.

4. A. Lilja, S. Hagstadius, J. Risberg, L. G. Salford, G. J. W. Smith, "Frontal lobe dynamics in brain tumor patients: a study of regional cerebral blood flow and affective changes before and after surgery," *J Neuropsychiatry Neuropsychol Behav Neurol* 5, vol (1992).

5. M. S. Nobler, H. A. Sakheim, I. Prohovnik, J. R. Moeller, S. Mukherjee, D. B. Schur J. Prudic, D. P. Devanand, "Regional cerebral blood flow in mood disorders: III. Treatment and clinical response," *Arch Gen Psychiatry* 51, no. 11 (1994): 884–897.

6. J. Risberg, "Regional cerebral blood flow measurements by ^{133}Xe-inhalation: methodology and applications in neuropsychology and psychiatry," *Brain Lang* 9, no. 1 (1980): 9–34.

7. W. G. Honer, I. Prohovnik, G. Smith, L. R. Lucas, "Scopolamine reduces frontal cortex perfusion," *J Cereb Blood Flow Metab* 8, no. 5 (1988): 635–641.

8. E. Goldberg, A. Kluger, T. Griesing, L. Malta, M. Shapiro, S. Ferris, "Early diagnosis of frontal-lobe dementias." Presented at the Eighth Congress of the International Psychogeriatric Association; August, 17–22, 1997; Jerusalem, Israel.

9. E. Goldberg, "Introduction: the frontal lobes in neurological and psychiatric conditions," *Neuropsychiatry Neuropsychol, Behav Neurol* 5, no. 4 (1992): 231–232.

10. J. H. Jackson, "Evolution and dissolution of the nervous system," *Croonian Lecture. Selected Papers* 2 (1884).

11. A. R. Luria, *Higher Cortical Functions in Man* (New York: Basic Books, 1966).

12. E. Goldberg and L. D. Costa, "Qualitative indices in neuropsychological assessment: an extension of Luria's approach to executive deficit following prefrontal lesion," in *Neuropsychological Assessment of Neuropsychiatric Disorders*, ed. I. Grant and K. M. Adams (New York: Oxford University Press, 1985), 48–64.

13. See K. Heilman and E. Valenstein, eds., *Clinical Neuropsychology* (New York: Oxford University Press, 1993).

14. E. Moniz, "Essai d'un traitement chirurgical de certaines psychoses," *Bull Acad Natl Med* 115 (1936): 385–392.

15. See K. Heilman and E. Valenstein, eds., Clinical Neuropsychology (New York: Oxford University Press, 1993).

16. Dr. Robert Iacono (personal communication), January 2000.

17. A. Ploghaus, I. Tracey, J. S. Gati, S. Clare, R. S. Menon, P. M. Matthews, J. N. Rawlings, "Dissociating pain from its anticipation in the human brain," *Science* 284, no. 5422 (1999): 1979–1981.

18. D. H. Ingvar, "'Memory of the future: an essay on the temporal organization of conscious awareness," *Hum Neurobiol* 4, no. 3 (1985): 127–136.

19. From E. Goldberg and L. D. Costa, "Qualitative indices in neuropsychological assessment: an extension of Luria's approach to executive deficit following prefrontal lesion," in *Neuropsychological Assessment of Neuropsychiatric Disorders*, ed. I. Grant and K. M. Adams (New York: Oxford University Press, 1985), 55.

20. F. Lhermitte, "Utilization behavior and its relationship to lesions of the frontal lobes," *Brain* 106 (1983): 237–255.

21. For more detailed description see M. D. Lezak, *Neuropsychological Assessment*, 3rd ed. (New York: Oxford University Press, 1995).

22. P. Goldman-Rakic (personal communication), February 1991.

23. K. Brodmann, "Neue Ergebnisse über die vergleichende histologische Lokalisation der Grosshirnrinde mit besonderer Berücksichtigung des Stirnhirns," *Anat Anz* 41 (1912; suppl): 157–216. Cited in J. M. Fuster, *The Prefrontal Cortex: Anatomy, Physiology, and Neuropsychology of the Frontal Lobe*, 3rd ed. (Philadelphia: Lippincott–Raven, 1997).

24. R. A. Barkley, *ADHD and the Nature of Self-Control* (New York: Guilford Press, 1997).

25. S. L. Rauch, M. A. Jenike, N. M. Alpert, L. Baer, H. G. Breiter, C. R. Savage, A. J. Fischman, "Regional cerebral blood flow measured during symp-

tom provocation in obsessive-compulsive disorder using oxygen 15–labeled carbon dioxide and positron emission tomography," *Arch Gen Psychiatry* 51, no. 1 (1994): 62–70.

26. A. R. Luria, *Higher Cortical Functions in Man* (New York: Basic Books, 1966).

27. E. Goldberg and D. Tucker, "Motor perseverations and long-term memory for visual forms," *J Clin Neuropsychol* 1, no. 4 (1979): 273–288.

28. D. A. Grant and E. A. Berg, "A behavioral analysis of degree of reinforcement and ease of shifting to new responses in a Weigl-type card-sorting problem," *J Exp Psychol* 38 (1948): 404–411.

29. For review see K. Heilman and E. Valenstein, eds., *Clinical Neuropsychology* (New York: Oxford University Press, 1993).

30. E. Goldberg and W. B. Barr, "Three possible mechanisms of unawareness deficit," in *Awareness of Deficit after Brain Injury*, ed. G. Prigatano and D. Schacter (New York: Oxford University Press, 1991), 152–175.

31. Ibid.

Chapter 9: Social Maturity, Morality, Law, and the Frontal Lobes

1. H. Oppenheim, "Zur Pathologie der Grosshirngeschwulste," *Arch Psychiatry* 21 (1889): 560.

2. A. Schore, *Affect Regulation and the Origin of the Self: The Neurobiology of Emotional Development* (Hillsdale, New Jersey: Lawrence Erlbaum Associates, 1999).

3. S. W. Anderson, A. Bechara, H. Damasio, D. Tranel, A. R. Damasio, "Impairment of social and moral behavior related to early damage in human prefrontal cortex," *Nat Neurosci* 2, no. 11 (1999): 1032–1037.

4. M. I. Posner and M. K. Rothbart, "Attention, self-regulation and consciousness," *Philos Trans R Soc Lond B Biol Sci* 353, no. 1377 (1998): 1915–1927.

5. P. I. Yakovlev and A. R. Lecours, "The myelogenetic cycles of regional maturation of the brain," in *Regional Development of the Brain in Early Life*, ed. A. Minkowski (Oxford: Blackwell 1967), 3–70.

6. W. Golding, *Lord of the Flies*, rpt (Mattituck, New York: Amereon House 1999).

7. J. Volavka, *Neurobiology of Violence* (Washington, DC: American Psychiatric Press, 1995); A. Raine, *The Psychopathology of Crime: Criminal Behavior as a Clinical Disorder* (San Diego: Academic Press, 1993).

8. E. Goldberg, R. M. Bilder, J. E. Hughes, S. P. Antin, S. Mattis, "A reticulo-frontal disconnection syndrome," *Cortex* 25, no. 4 (1989): 687–695.

9. A. Raine, M. Buchsbaum, and L. LaCasse, "Brain abnormalities in murderers indicated by positron emission tomography," *Biol Psychiatry* 42, no. 6 (1997): 495–508.

10. A. Raine, T. Lencz, S. Bihrle, L. LaCasse, P. Colletti, "Reduced prefrontal gray matter volume and reduced autonomic activity in antisocial personality disorder," *Arch Gen Psychiatry* 57, no. 2 (2000): 119–127; discussion 128–129.

11. A. R. Luria, *Higher Cortical Functions in Man* (New York: Basic Books, 1966).

12. E. Goldberg, K. Podell, R. Bilder, J. Jaeger, "The executive control battery," *Psych Press* (Australia: 2000); E. Goldberg, K. Podell, R. Bilder, J. Jaeger, "Test for bedomning av exekutive dysfunktion," *Psykologiforlaget AB* (Sweden: 1997).

13. For test description see M. D. Lezak, *Neuropsychological Assessment*, 3rd ed. (New York: Oxford University Press, 1995).

14. O. W. Sacks, *The Man Who Mistook His Wife for a Hat: And Other Clinical Tales* (New York: Touchstone Books, 1998).

Chapter 10: Fateful Disconnections

1. N. Geshwind, "Disconnexion syndromes in animals and man," *Brain* 88 (1965): 237–294.

2. E. Goldberg, R. M. Bilder, J. E. Hughes, S. P. Antin, S. Mattis, "A reticulo-frontal disconnection syndrome," *Cortex* 25, no. 4 (1989): 687–695.

3. E. Goldberg, S. P. Antin, R. M. Bilder Jr., L. J. Gerstman, J. E. Hughes, S. Mattis, "Retrograde amnesia: possible role of mesencephalic reticular activation in long-term memory," *Science* 213, no. 4514 (1981): 1392–1394.

4. For review see H. S. Nasrallah, ed., *Handbook of Schizophrenia* (New York: Elsevier, 1991).

5. E. Kraepelin, *Dementia Praecox and Paraphrenia* (Edinburgh: E. S Livingstone, 1919/1971), vol. 4, p. 219.

6. K. F. Berman, R. F. Zec, and D. R. Weinberger, "Physiologic dysfunction of dorsolateral prefrontal cortex in schizophrenia: II. Role of neuroleptic treatment, attention, and mental effort," *Arch Gen Psychiatry* 43, no. 2 (1986): 126–135; D. R. Weinberger, K. F. Berman, and R. F. Zec, "Physiologic dysfunction of dorsolateral prefrontal cortex in schizophrenia: I. Regional cerebral blood flow evidence," *Arch Gen Psychiatry* 43, no. 2 (1986): 114–124.

7. B. Milner, "Effects of different brain lesions in card sorting: the role of the frontal lobes," *Arch Neurol* 9 (1963): 100–110; D. R. Weinberger, K. F. Berman, and R. F. Zec, "Physiologic dysfunction of dorsolateral prefrontal cortex in schizophrenia: I. Regional cerebral blood flow evidence," *Arch Gen Psychiatry* 43, no. 2 (1986): 114–124.

8. G. Franzen and D. H. Ingvar, "Absence of activation in frontal structures during psychological testing of chronic schizophrenics," *J Neurol Neurosurg Psychiatry* 38, no. 10 (1975): 1027–1032; M. S. Buchsbaum, L. E. DeLisi, H. H. Holcomb, J. Cappelletti, A. C. King, J. Johnson, E. Hazlett, S. Dowling-Zimmerman, R. M. Post, J. Morihisa, "Anteroposterior gradients in cerebral glucose use in schizophrenia and affective disorders," *Arch Gen Psychiatry* 41, no. 12 (1984): 1159–1166.

9. D. R. Weinberger and K. F. Berman, "Speculation on the meaning of cerebral metabolic hypofrontality in schizophrenia," *Schizophr Bull* 14, no. 2 (1988): 157–168.

10. E. Valenstein, *The Great and Desperate Cures* (New York: Basic Books, 1986).

11. J. R. Stevens, "An anatomy of schizophrenia?" *Arch Gen Psychiatry* 29, no. 2 (1973): 177–189; S. Matthysse, "Dopamine and the pharmacology of schizophrenia: the state of the evidence," *J Psychiatr Res* 11 (1974): 107–113.

12. For review see J. R. Cooper, F. E. Bloom, and R. H. Roth, *The Biochemical Basis of Neuropharmacology*, 7th ed. (New York: Oxford University Press, 1996).

13. M. Carlsson and A. Carlsson, "Schizophrenia: a subcortical neurotransmitter imbalance syndrome?" *Schizophr Bull* 16, no. 3 (1990): 425–432.

14. For review see J. R. Cooper, F. E. Bloom, and R. H. Roth, *The Biochemical Basis of Neuropharmacology*, 7th ed. (New York: Oxford University Press, 1996).

15. E. S. Gershon and R. O. Rieder, "Major disorders of mind and brain," *Sci Am* 267, no. 3 (1992): 126–133.

16. B. Kolb and I. Q. Whishaw, *Fundamentals of Human Neuropsychology*, 4th ed. (New York: WH Freeman & Co, 1995).

17. National Institute of Neurological Disorders and Stroke, *Interagency Head Injury Task Force Report* (Bethesda, Maryland: National Institutes of Health, 1989).

18. J. C. Masdeu, H. Abdel-Dayem, and R. L. Van Heertum, "Head trauma: use of SPECT," *J Neuroimaging* 5 (1995; suppl 1): S53–57.

19. E. Goldberg and D. Bougakov, "Novel approaches to the diagnosis and treatment of frontal lobe dysfunction," in *International Handbook of Neuropsychological Rehabilitation*, eds. A.-L. Christensen and B. P. Uzzel (New York: Kluwer Academic/Plenum Publishers, 2000), 93–112.

20. Ibid.

21. R. A. Barkley, *ADHD and the Nature of Self-Control* (New York: The Guilford Press, 1997).

22. From *Possible Poetry*, Toby's unpublished collection of poems written as a teenager on the streets of Sydney. Reprinted with the author's permission.

23. G. G. Tourette, "Étude sur une affection nerveuse caractérisée par de l'incoordination motrice accompagnée d'écholalie et de copralalie," *Arch Neurol* 9 (1885).

24. C. W. Bazil, "Seizures in the life and works of Edgar Allan Poe," *Arch Neurol* 56, no. 6 (1999): 740–743; E. A. Poe, *The Complete Tales and Poems of Edgar Allan Poe* (New York: Barnes & Noble Books, 1989).

25. E. Shapiro, A. K. Shapiro, and J. Clarkin, "Clinical psychological testing in Tourette's syndrome," *J Pers Assess* 38, no. 5 (1974): 464–478.

26. D. M. Sheppard, J. L. Bradshaw, R. Purcell, C. Pantelis, "Tourette's and comorbid syndromes: obsessive compulsive and attention deficit hyperactivity disorder. A common etiology?" *Clin Psychol Rev* 19, no. 5 (1999): 531–552.

27. O. W. Sacks, "Tourette's syndrome and creativity," *Br Med J* 305 (1992): 1515–1516.

28. L. Handler, *Twitch and Shout: A Touretter's* Tale (New York: Plume, 1999).

Chapter 11: "What Can You Do for Me?"

1. E. Goldberg, L. J. Gerstman, S. Mattis, J. E. Hughes, C. A. Sirio, R. M. Bilder Jr., "Selective effects of cholinergic treatment on verbal memory in posttraumatic amnesia," *J Clin Neuropsychol* 4, no. 3 (1982): 219–234.

2. V. M. Polyakov, L. I. Moskovichyute, and E. G. Simernitskaya, "Neuropsychological analysis of the role in brain functional organization in man," in *Modern Problems in Neurobiology*, ed. (Tbilisi: 1986), 329–330; O. A. Krotkova, T. A. Karaseva, and L. I. Moskovichyute, "Lateralization features of the dynamics of higher mental functions following endonasal glutamic acid electrophoresis," *Zh Vopr Neirokhir Im N N Burdenko*, no. 3 (1982): 48–52; N. K. Korsakova and L. I. Moskovichyute, *Subcortical Structures and Psychological Processes* (Moscow: Moscow University Publishing House, 1985); L. I. Moskovitchyute, M. Mimura, and M. Albert, "Selective effect of dopamine on apraxia." Presented at the AAN Annual Meeting, May 1–7, 1994, Washington, D.C.

3. B. H. Dobkin and R. Hanlon, "Dopamine agonist treatment of anterograde amnesia from a mediobasal forebrain injury," *Ann Neurol* 33, no. 3 (1993): 313–316.

4. D. E. Hobson, E. Pourcher, and W. R. Martin, "Ropinirole and pramipexole, the new agonists," *Can J Neurol Sci* 26 (1999; suppl 2): S27–33.

5. E. D. Ross and R. M. Stewart, "Akinetic mutism from hypothalamic damage: successful treatment with dopamine agonists," *Neurology* 31 (1981): 1435–1439; B. H. Dobkin and R. Hanlon, "Dopamine agonist treatment of antegrade amnesia from a mediobasal forebrain injury," *Ann Neurol* 33, no. 3 (1993): 313–316.

6. M. F. Kraus and P. Maki, "The combined use of amantadine and L-dopa/carbidopa in the treatment of chronic brain injury," *Brain Inj* 11, no. 6 (1997): 455–460; M. F. Kraus and P. M. Maki, "Effect of amantadine hydrochloride on symptoms of frontal lobe dysfunction in brain injury: case studies and review," *J Neuropsychiatry Clin Neurosci* 9, no. 2 (1997): 222–230.

7. D. Golden, "Building a better brain," *Life*, July 1994, 62–70.

8. A. Damasio, *Descartes' Error: Emotion, Reason, and the Human Brain* (New York: Putnam Publishing Group, 1994); A. Damasio, *The Feeling of What Happens: Body and Emotion in the Making of Consciousness* (New York: Harcourt Brace, 1999).

9. J. W. Rowe and R. L. Kahn, *Successful Aging* (New York: Pantheon, 1998).

10. R. Katzman, "The prevalence and malignancy of Alzheimer's disease: a major killer," *Arch Neurol* 33 (1976): 217.

11. A. Newell and H. A. Simon, *Human Problem Solving* (Englewood Cliffs, New Jersey: Prentice-Hall, 1972); H. A. Simon, P. Langley, G. Bradshaw, J. Zykow, *Scientific Discovery: Exploration of the Creative Process* (Cambridge: MIT Press, 1987).

12. R. J. Hamm, M. D. Temple, D. M. O'Dell, B. R. Pike, B. G. Lyeth, "Exposure to environmental complexity promotes recovery of cognitive function after traumatic brain injury," *J Neurotrauma* 13, no. 1 (1996): 41–47.

13. B. Kolb, *Brain Plasticity and Behavior* (Mahwah, New Jersey: Lawrence Erlbaum Associates, 1995).

14. W. D. Heiss, J. Kessler, R. Mielke, B. Szelies, K. Herholtz, "Long-term effects of phosphatidylserine, pyritinol, and cognitive training in Alzheimer's disease: a neuropsychological, EEG, and PET investigation," *Dementia* 5, no. 2 (1994): 88–98.

15. E. Gould, P. Tanapat, B. S. McEwen, G. Flugge, E. Fuchs, "Proliferation of granule cell precursors in the dentate gyrus of adult monkeys is diminished by stress," *Proc Natl Acad Sci U S A* 95, no. 6 (1998): 3168–3171.

16. E. Gould, A. J. Reeves, M. S. Graziano, C. G. Gross, "Neurogenesis in the neocortex of adult primates," *Science* 286, no. 5439 (1999): 548–552.

17. G. Kempermann, H. G. Kuhn, and F. H. Gage, "More hippocampal neurons in adult mice living in an enriched environment," *Nature* 386, no. 6624 (1997): 493–495.

18. Ibid.

19. Ibid.

20. M. S. Albert, K. Jones, C. R. Savage, L. Berkman, T. Seeman, D. Blazer, J. W. Rowe, "Predictors of cognitive change in older persons: MacArthur studies of successful aging," *Psychol Aging* 10, no. 4 (1995): 578–589.

21. D. A. Snowdon, S. J. Kemper, J. A. Mortimer, L. H. Greiner, D. R. Wekstein, W. R. Markesbery, "Linguistic ability in early life and cognitive function and Alzheimer's disease in late life: findings from the Nun Study [see comments]," *Jama* 275, no. 7 (1996): 528–532.

22. Ibid.

23. F. Dellu, W. Mayo, M. Valee, M. Le Moaz, H. Simon, "Facilitation of cognitive performance in aged rats by past experience depends on the type of information processing involved: a combined cross-sectional and longitudinal study," *Neurobiol Learn Mem* 67, no. 2 (1997): 121–128.

24. K. W. Schaie and S. L. Willis, "Can decline in adult intellectual functioning be reversed?" *Dev Psychol* 22, no. 2 (1986): 223.

25. W. D. Heiss, J. Kessler, R. Mielke, B. Szelies, K. Herholz, "Long-term effects of phosphatidylserine, pyritinol, and cognitive training in Alzheimer's disease: a neuropsychological, EEG, and PET investigation," *Dementia* 5, no. 2 (1994): 88–98.

26. M. Mirmiran, E. J. van Someren, and D. F. Swaab, "Is brain plasticity preserved during aging and in Alzheimer's disease?" *Behav Brain Res* 78, no. 1 (1996): 43–48.

27. E. A. Maguire, D. G. Gadian, I. S. Johnsrude, C. D. Good, J. Ashburner, R. S. Frakowiak, C. D. Frith, "Navigation-related structural change in the hippocampi of taxi drivers," *Proc Natl Acad Sci U S A* 97, no. 8 (2000): 4398–4403.

28. B. L. McNaughton, "Associative pattern competition in hippocampal circuits: new evidence and new questions," *Brain Res Rev* 16 (1991): 202–204; B. L. McNaughton and R. G. M Morris, "Hippocampal synaptic enhancement and information storage," *Trends Neurosci* 10 (1987): 408–415.

Chapter 12: Frontal Lobes and the Leadership Paradox

1. J. A. Fodor, "Precis of the modularity of mind," *Behav Brain Sci* 8 (1985): 1–42.

2. E. Goldberg, "Gradiental approach to neocortical functional organization," *J Clin Exp Neuropsychol* 11, no. 4 (1989): 489–517; E. Goldberg, "Higher cortical functions in humans: the gradiental approach," in *Contemporary Neuropsychology and the Legacy of Luria*, ed. E. Goldberg (Hillsdale, New Jersey:

Lawrence Erlbaum Associates, 1990), 229–276; E. Goldberg, "Rise and fall of modular orthodoxy," *J Clin Exp Neuropsychol* 17, no. 2 (1995): 193–208.

3. W. S. McCulloch and W. Pitts, "A logical calculus of the ideas immanent in nervous activity. 1943 classical article," *Bull Math Biol* 52, no. 1–2 (1990): 99–115.

4. E. Goldberg, "Gradiental approach to neocortical functional organization," *J Clin Exp Neuropsychol* 11, no. 4 (1989): 489–517.

5. D. Oakley and H. Plotkin, eds., *Brain, Behavior and Evolution* (Cambridge, UK: Cambridge University Press, 1979).

6. S. Nunn and A. N. Stulberg, "The many faces of modern Russia," *Foreign Affairs* 79, no. 2 (2000): 45–62.

7. M. Simons, "In new Europe, a lingual hodgepodge," *The New York Times,* October 17 1999, A4.

8. K. Ohmae, *The End of the Nation State: The Rise of Regional Economies* (New York: Free Press, 1995).

9. P. Lewis, "As nations shed roles, is medieval the future?" *The New York Times,* January 2, 1999, B7, B9.

10. R. D. Kaplan, *Coming Anarchy: Shattering the Dreams of the Post Cold War* (New York: Random House, 2000).

11. S. J. Kobrin, "Back to the future: neo-medievalism and post-modern digital world," *Journal of International Affairs* 51, no. 2 (1998): 361–386.

12. W. S. McCulloch and W. Pitts, "A logical calculus of the ideas immanent in nervous activity: 1943 classical article," *Bull Math Biol* 52, no. 1–2 (1990): 99–115.

13. R. D. Kaplan, *Coming Anarchy: Shattering the Dreams of the Post Cold War* (New York: Random House, 2000).

14. E. D. Tucker, ed., *The Marx-Engels Reader,* 2nd ed. (New York: W W Norton, 1978). As an ideological slogan in the old Soviet Union, this phrase acquired a distinctly sadistic twist, vaguely akin to "Arbeit Macht Frei" (German for "work liberates," a sign on the gates of Auschwitz). In 1968, the year of the suppressed Prague Spring, a grim joke circulated around Moscow, that then president of Czechoslovakia General Svoboda ("svoboda" meaning "freedom" in Russian) had been renamed General Poznannaya Neobhodimostj ("General Recognized Necessity").

Epilogue

1. B. Spinoza, *Ethics,* trans. A. Boyle (London: Everyman, 1997).

2. Ibid.

3. W. S. McCulloch and W. Pitts, "A logical calculus of the ideas immanent in nervous activity: 1943 classical article," *Bull Math Biol* 52, no. 1–2 (1990): 99–115.

4. W. Pitts and W. S. McCulloch, "How we know universals: the perception of auditory and visual forms," *Bull Math Biophys* 9 (1947): 127–147.

Index

Acetylcholine. *See* Neurotransmitter
Acquired immunodeficiency syndrome, 5–6, 167
Actor-centered decision making. *See* Frontal lobes and adaptive decision making
ADD. *See* Attention deficit disorder
ADHD. *See* Attention deficit hyperactivity disorder
Agnosia. *See* Gradiental principle and "associative agnosias"
AIDS. *See* Acquired immunodeficiency syndrome
Altman, J., 206
Alzheimer's disease, 6, 83–85,113–115, 167, 194–196, 198, 205, 208, 211–212
  and cognitive exercise and the "nun" study, 208–209
  pharmacological treatment of, 194–196
  statistics of, 199
Anosognosia, 135–137
Anticholinesterases. *See* Alzheimer's disease, pharmacological treatment of
Aphasia, 41
ARAS. *See* Ascending reticular activating system
Ascending reticular activating system (ARAS), 29, 161. *See also* Attention deficit hyperactivity disorder as dysfunction in frontal-reticular-posterior cortical attentional loop
Attention deficit disorder (ADD), 4, 6, 103, 114, 168–173
  as social phenomenon, 169
Attention deficit hyperactivity disorder (ADHD), 4, 96, 129, 168–173
  case study of, 173–180
  as dysfunction in frontal-reticular-posterior cortical attentional loop, 171–173
Autism, 103

Benson, F., 35
Bernstein, N., 9
Brain structure. *See also* Gradiental principle of brain organization; Modularity
  cellular, 27–29
  and complexity, 27–28, 217–219
  gross-anatomical, 29–35
    amygdala, 31, 36
    basal ganglia, 30, 35
    brain stem, 29, 36
    caudate nuclei, 30
    cerebellum, 31, 35
    cingulate cortex, 31, 36
    diencephalon, 30
    dorsomedial thalamic nucleus, 34, 36
    hippocampus, 31, 36
    globus pallidus, 30, 31
    hypothalamus, 30, 36
    metaphor of a tree, 29

Brain structure (*continued*)
nuclei and regions, 29
putamen, 30
thalamus, 30, 36
plasticity over the life span, 206
region size and environmental factors, 212
Brodmann, K., 33
Brodmann areas, 33, 34f
Broca, P., 41
Bull, H., 223

Cartesian dualism, 2, 155
CBT. *See* Cognitive Bias Task
CEO. *See* Chief executive officer
Chief executive officer (CEO), and role of a leader, 21–22, 78
Cognitive Bias Task (CBT), 79–80
and Alzheimer's-type dementia, 83–85, 84f
and brain damage, 95–97
and gender differences in decision-making, 89–93, 90f, 95–97
and handedness, 99, 101, 103
and influence of lesion site on performance, 80–82, 82f
stimulus card, 81f
Cognitive fitness
history and modern trends of, 200–202
Cognitive exercise. *See also* Alzheimer's disease and cognitive exercise and the "nun" study
and effects of on brain glucose metabolism, 210
and neurostimulant medication, 205
and neuronal proliferation, 207
Cognitive fitness
concept of, 210–212
working model of, 212–214
Cognitive rehabilitation,
and "functional system" concept, 203
and effects of treatment of brain damage, 210
"Cognotropic" pharmacology, 6, 168, 194–197
Coleman, D., 105
Complexity, 219–223. *See also* Brain structure and complexity and geopolitical trends
Coprolalia, 183
Cortical areas involved in drawing to dictation, 131f
Costa, L., 43
Courtney, S., 76
Creativity and mental illness, 181
"Creation of Adam" by Michelangelo, and the brain, 24
Cytoarchitectonic regions and/or maps, 32, 33

Damasio, A., 35, 142, 197
and "Descartes' error," 2, 114
Dellu, F., 209
Dementia, 5, 6, 198–200. *See also* Azheimer's disease
and education, 207–209
Descartes, R., 228
Dichotic studies, 48
Disconnection syndrome, 160
Dopaminergic agonists
and mild traumatic brain injury and executive functions, 195–197
Dynamic topology, 218
Dyslexia, 103

Echolalia, 126
Echopraxia, 126
ECT. *See* Electroconvulsive shock
Electroconvulsive shock (ECT), 43
Engels, F., 226
Executive control battery, 149
Executive functions. *See* Frontal lobes, function of and "smartness," 106

Field-dependent behavior, 125–126
Frontal lobes. *See also* Prefrontal cortex
and adaptive decision making, 77–79, 93. *See also* Cognitive Bias Task
and Alzheimer's disease, 115
biological vulnerability of, 114–116
and neuroimaging data, 114–115
as chief executive officer (CEO) metaphor, 24–26
as cortical constraining factor, 218
and dorsolateral syndrome, 117–118, 139
and lobotomy, 117–118
case studies, 118–126, 130–135

and gender differences in decision-making
and Cognitive Bias Task (CBT), 79–83, 95
in brain damage, 95–97
function of, 24–26
and language, 25
maturity of
and distress regulation, 142–143
and morality and criminal behavior, 141–143, 146–149
and rights of passage, 143–146
and "memory of the future," 123–124, 127–129
and novelty, 69–71
and neuroimaging data, 69–71
familiarization effect, 70f, 71f
and orbitofrontal syndrome, 117, 139–141
case studies, 150–155
and search engine analogy, 225–226
and self–nonself discrimination, 110–112
and smartness, 106
and theory of mind, 108
in brain pathology, 109–110
Frontal lobe ratio to the whole brain, 33f
Frontal-reticular-posterior cortical attentional loop, 172f
Functional neuroimaging
limitations of, 54–55
Fuster, J., 35, 74

Gall, F. J., 37, 39–40, 55
and phrenological maps, 37–40, 38f
Gardner, M., 105
Gates, B., 202
Geshwind, N., 160
"G-factor" and "multiple intelligences," 105–106
Gold, J., 50, 71
Goldman-Rakic, P., 35, 74, 77, 127
Gould, E., 206
Gradiental principle
and "associative agnosias," 62–64
of brain organization, 215–219
and digital world, 224–226
and knowledge representation, 64–67
Grossberg, S., 45

Handedness
and cognitive styles, 101
in humans vs. animals, 101
and left-handedness and creativity, 101, 104
and mental disorder, 103–104
Head trauma, 4. *See also* Traumatic brain injury
Hemispheric specialization
and anosognosia, 136–137
and cognitive "landscapes," 52–55
and cognitive novelty vs. cognitive routinization, 43–52
and brain acivation as a function of task familiarization, 49f
and music, 47–48
and neural nets, 45
and neuroimaging evidence 47–52
and prosapognosia, 47–48
tachisoscopic and dichotic studies, 48
and hemispheric asymmetries, 41
in apes, 42
and brain biochemistry, 42, 94
in brain pathology, 96
and gender differences, 41, 94–95, 98. *See also* Frontal lobes and adaptive decision making
in brain damage
and language, 41–43, 45
and planum temporale and sylvian fissure, 41, 42

Iacono, R., 118
Ingvar, D., 123

Jacobsen, C., 73
Jackson, H., 35, 74, 115
Jaynes, J.
and prefrontal cortex and voices of god, 23, 52
and self–nonself discrimination, 111–112

Kaplan, R., 223, 224
Kleist, K., 39–40
and cortical maps, 39–40, 39f
Korbin, S., 223
Kraepelin, E., 163

Language
distribute cortical representation of, 66f
Leontyev, A., 8
Lewis, P., 222
Lewy body disease, 205, 211
Limbic system, 31
Luria, A. R, 2, 4, 7–11, 10f, 15–17, 19, 35, 42, 61, 73, 198, 203, 228–229
Lana Pimenovna, 10, 11, 17,19
Lena, 16
Lysenko, T., 204

Martin, A., 49, 65
Masdeu, J., 167
McCulloch, W., 223, 229
McEwen, B., 206
Meier-Graefe, J., 24
Memory
as a metaphor, 5
frontal lobes and working, 72–77
Moniz, E., 117
Mishkin, M., 99, 102
Modularity, 55–58, 62, 64, 215–219
and digital world, 224–226
and "strong dissociations," 56

Neocortex
evolutionary advantage of, 217–219
organization of, 32–33, 58
and "cognitive gradients," 59, 61–67
and gender diffrences, 97–98
Neural nets. *See also* Hemispheric specialization, and cognitive novelty vs. cognitive routinization, and neural nets
and brain models, 216
and cognitive gender differences, 98
and digital world, 225
Neurotransmitter
acetylcholine, 28
dopamine, 28, 35, 42, 103, 161, 165–166, 182, 196
gamma-aminobutyric acid (GABA), 28, 165–166
glutamate, 28, 165–166
norepinephrine, 28, 42
serotonin, 28
Nottebohm, F., 206
Novelty seeking behavior
and acquired vs. inherited knowledge
in monkeys, 99–100, 102
and handedness, 102
in humans, 99–100, 103

Obsessive-compulsive disorder (OCD), 4, 114, 130
Ohmae, K., 222

Perseveration, 131–134
and inertia of termination, 120f
variety of, 132f
Pick's disease, 149, 205
Pitts, W., 223, 229
Posner, M., 54, 142–143
Prefrontal cortex, 35f. *See also* Frontal lobes
connections of, 35–36
and consciousness, 36
ratio of, across evolution, 33
structural definition of, 33–35
Pribram, K., 99
Principle of double dissociation, 53

Raichle, M., 51, 69
Raine, A., 147
Reagan, R., 199
Reticulofrontal disconnection syndrome
schematic drawing of, 162
case study of, 157–163
mechanism of, 161, 168
Risberg, J., 114–115

Sacks, O., 62, 156, 183–185
Schaei, W., 209
Scheibel, A., 205
Schore, A., 141
Schizophrenia, 4, 5, 96, 103, 113–114, 120, 129, 163–164, 167
biochemical mechanisms of, 165–166
and neuroimaging correlates of positive and negative symptoms, 164
Simon, H., 43
Sontag, S., 5
Spinoza, B., 228–229
Stroop Test, 126–127
Stuss, D., 35
Swaab, D., 212

Tachistopic studies, 48
Tailarach space, 87–88
TBI. *See* Traumatic brain injury
Tilney, F., 23
Theory of mind, 107–108
  and frontal lobes, 108–112
Traumatic brain injury (TBI)
  and frontal dysfunction in absence of frontal lesion, 167–168
    and "cognotropic" pharmacology, 168, 196–197
    and neuroimaging evidence of hypofrontality, 167–168
  and animal recovery in enriched vs. ordinary environment
  statistics of, 167
Tourette's syndrome, 4, 96, 114, 180–192
  comorbidity of, 184
  mechanisms of, 182–184
  and patient's point of view, 185–192
  pictures of people with, 186
  symptoms of, 180–184
Tulving, E., 51

Vygotsky, L., 9

Weinberger, D., 164
Wernicke, K., 41
Willis, S., 209
Wisconsin Card Sorting Test, 135, 164
Witzelsucht, 140
Working memory, 73–77
  role of prefrontal cortex in, 76–77

Yakovlev, P., 41
Yakovlevian torque, 41, 94